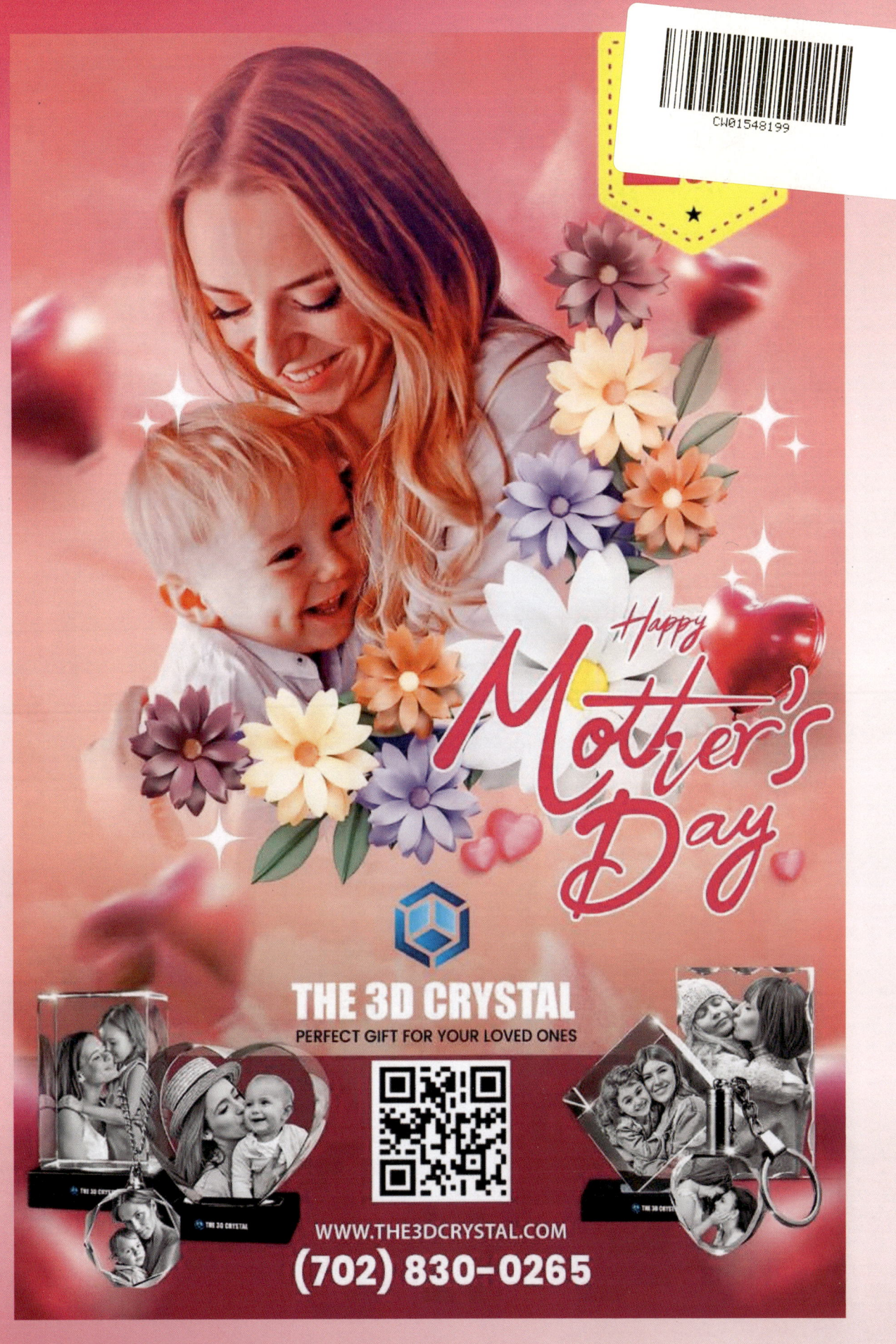

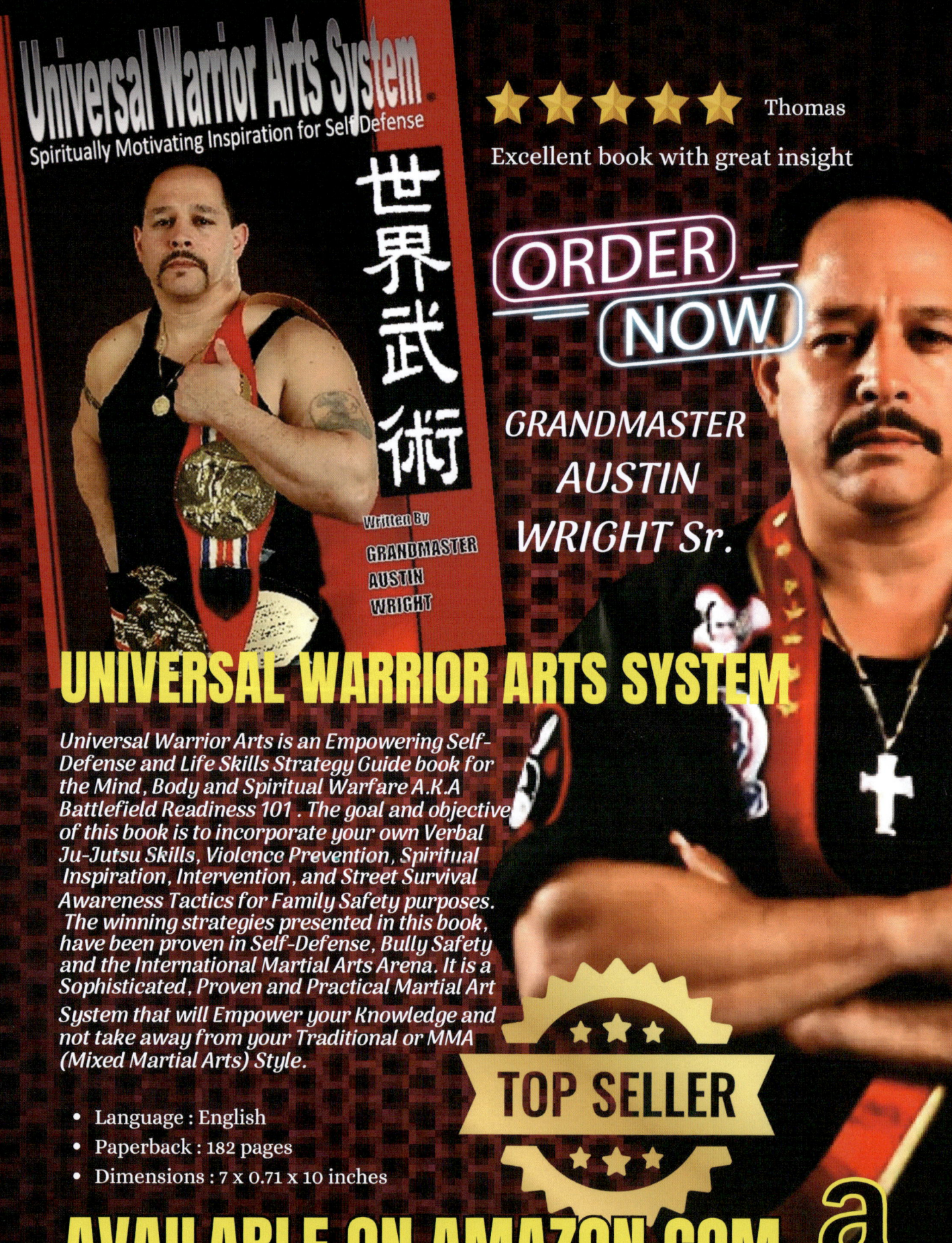

SANDOKAN
The Cutting Edge Martial Art

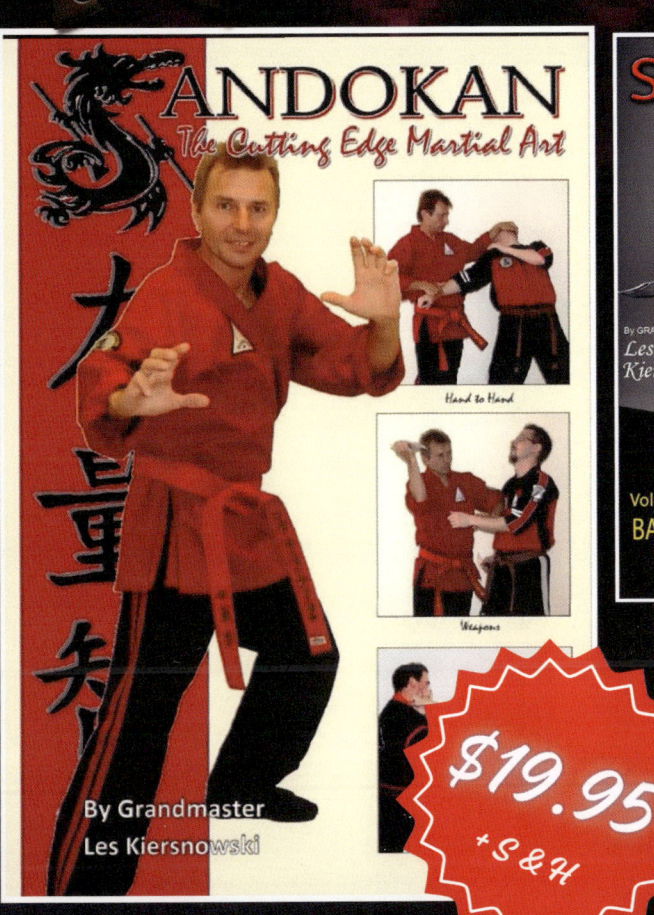

Basic Street Knife Defense DVD 1 $19.95

Tactical Knife Disarms & Control DVD 2 $19.95

Combative Double Blade Drills & Forms DVD 3 $19.95

$19.95 +S&H

The Sandokan system is based on physics, principles of martial science, and the science of anatomy. Achieving this martial arts system has encompassed many years of research and practical development. It is a system based on the perfecting of body positioning for maximum output of energy.

293 pages   English   2019   7 x 0.66 x 10 inch

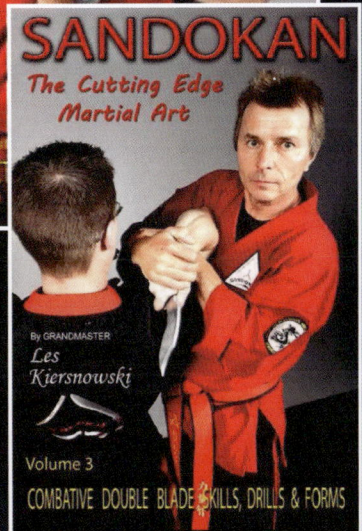

ORDER NOW

AVAILABLE ON AMAZON.COM

AVAILABLE NOW

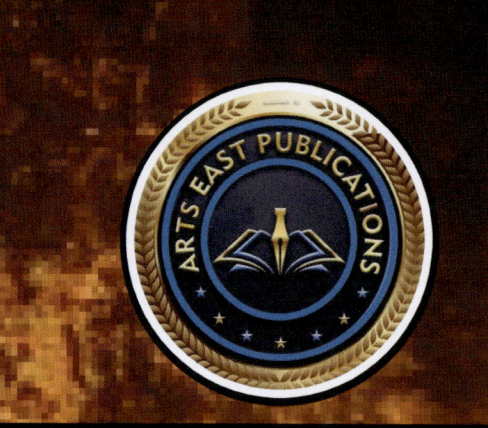
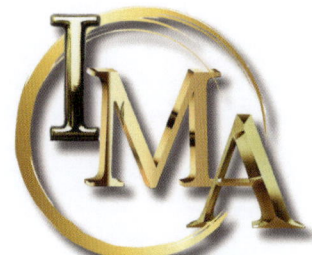

TABLE OF Contents
INTERNATIONAL MARTIAL ARTS MAGAZINE

Editor in Chief
Allen Woodman

Executive VP
Sumiko Nakano

Contributors
Joseph Miller
Cynthia Rothrock
Frank Dux
Gloria Hendry
Gary Dill
Sumiko Nakano
Allen Woodman
Paul Casey
Jim Arvanitis
Michelle Manu

Photographers
Mario Prado
Kim Marra

Assistant Editor
Sumiko Nakano

Creative Design
Allen Woodman

Social Media Coordinator
Lynn Holder

Marketing / Sales
Allen Woodman
Sumiko Nakano
Lynn Holder

7	**Editorial** — Allen Woodman
9	**PUT UP YOUR DUX** — Frank Dux
12	**THE HEALING TOUCH** — Joe MIller
14	**JKD The Old Way** — Gary Dill
19	**WOMEN WARRIORS** — GLORIA HENDRY BUNNY TO BOND GIRL — Sumiko Nakano & Allen Woodman
26	**FEATURED ARTICLE** — CYNTHIA ROTHROCK FRESH FROM BLACK CREEK — Sumiko Nakano
34	**GENDER MATTERS** — Recovery in Martial Arts Women Are Not Small Men — Michelle Manu
40	**NATIONAL TOURNAMENT HIT HARD** — Allen Woodman
43	**PANKRATION PAR T 6** — Jim Arvanitis
48	**KENPO CORNER** — Paul Casey
52	**ECHOES IN THE DOJO** — RICHARD NORTON A LIFE WELL LIVED — Allen Woodman
58	**GRAND OPENING** — Keith McCrary

May 2025 / Vol. 2 - No. 5

ABOUT THE COVER

On the cover of this month's issue of
INTERNATIONAL MARTIAL ARTS MAGAZINE
CYNTHIA ROTHROCK

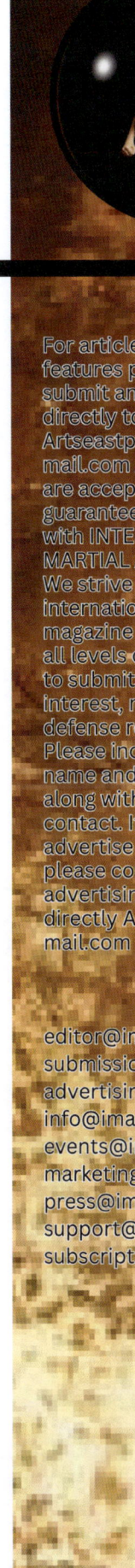

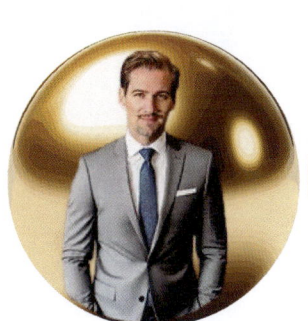
Editor In Chief
Allen Woodman

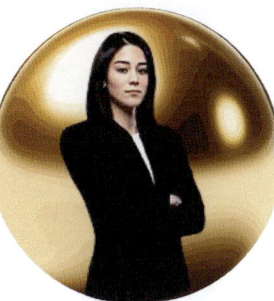
Excutive V.P.
Sumiko Nakano

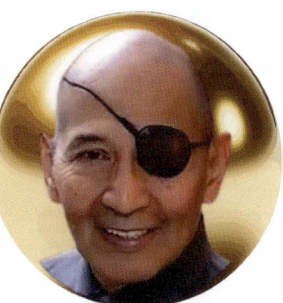
Photographer
Mario Prado

ARTS EAST Publications is the sole owner/manager of International Martial Arts Magazine © 2025

In the professional capacity of INTERNATIONAL MARTIAL ARTS MAGAZINE (hereinafter referred to as "IMAM"), it is hereby clarified that the copyrights and provisions concerning publisher indemnification pertinent to the articles published within IMAM are extensively governed by the following declarations:

IMAM expressly disclaims any responsibility or liability for the content of columns or articles authored by independent columnists, including, but not limited to, the techniques and methodologies delineated therein. The publication of any article within IMAM does not constitute an endorsement of its content.

All articles submitted and subsequently published in IMAM are done so with the full and discernible rights attributed to the respective author(s), under the principle that authorship confers exclusive copyright to the creator, unless explicitly stated otherwise in a contractual arrangement.

The engagement, practice, or training of any techniques, exercises, or movements demonstrated or advised within the scope of IMAM's published content is to be undertaken at the individual's discretion and risk. IMAM, inclusive of its publishers, editors, and contributors, assumes no liability for any injuries, damages, or other physical or psychological harm that may result from such endeavours.

Readers are advised to approach the replication of any demonstrated techniques with caution and to consult with professional instructors or healthcare providers before embarking on any physical training or martial arts program highlighted within IMAM's publications. This statement is intended to provide clarity on the legal and professional stance of IMAM regarding copyright, content liability, and the assumption of risk by its readership. IMAM remains dedicated to the dissemination of martial arts knowledge and culture, within the bounds of these defined terms.

For articles, columns or features please feel free to submit any written works directly to Artseastpublish@gmail.com All submissions are accepted by not guaranteed publication with INTERNATIONAL MARTIAL ARTS MAGAZINE. We strive for a true international input into our magazine and encourage all levels of practitioners to submit on any relevant interest, martial arts, self-defense related material. Please include authors full name and brief biography along with return email for contact. If you care to advertise with IMAM please contact our advertising department directly Artseastpublish@gmail.com

editor@imamag.org
submissions@imamag.org
advertising@imamag.org
info@imamag.org
events@imamag.org
marketing@imamag.org
press@imamag.org
support@imamag.org
subscriptions@imamag.org

May 2025 / Vol. 2 - No. 5

INTERNATIONAL MARTIAL ARTS INSTRUCTORS GUIDE 2025

BE A PART OF HISTORY IN THE MAKING

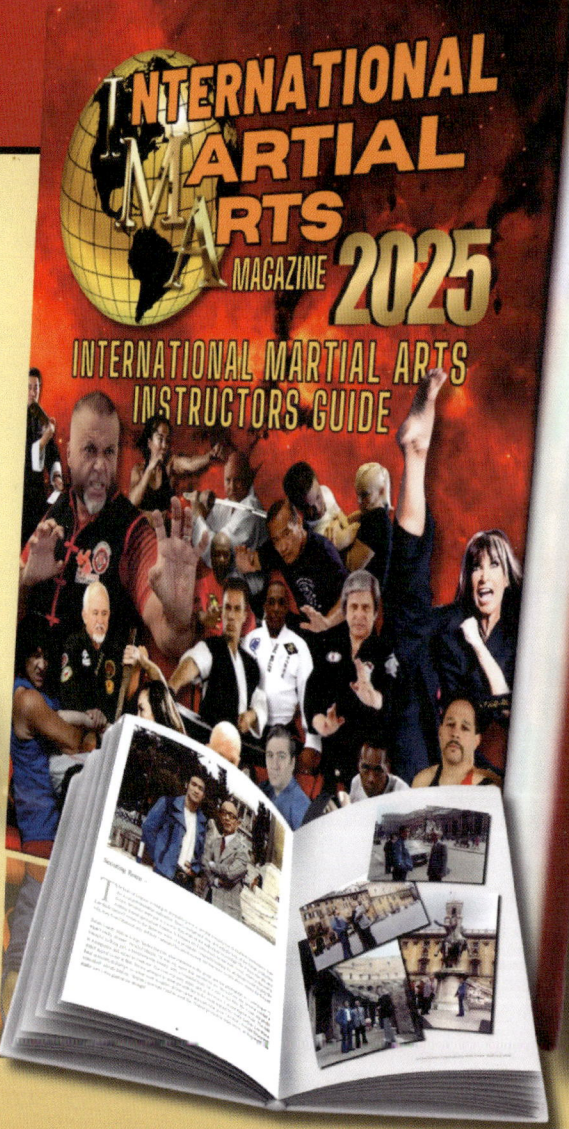

Submit Your Biography for the International Martial Arts Instructors Guide 2025! Attention all martial artists and instructors! Are you ready to showcase your skills and achievements to the world? Now is your chance! We are thrilled to announce the upcoming release of the International Martial Arts Instructors Guide 2025, a comprehensive volume dedicated to honoring the incredible talent and dedication found within the global martial arts community.

Why You Should Submit Your Biography This is more than just a book; it's a celebration of the rich tapestry of martial arts! Spanning over *300 pages*, this guide will feature profiles of practitioners from various styles and systems, making it the ultimate "who's who" in martial arts.

Whether you're a seasoned black belt or an emerging instructor, your story deserves to be told!

This is your opportunity to shine without any financial burden. - Global Exposure: Your biography will be seen by martial arts enthusiasts, practitioners, and instructors worldwide. -

High-Quality Presentation The guide will be printed in hardbound and paperback, featuring stunning full-color pages that bring your achievements to life.

We invite all martial artists, regardless of style—karate, judo, taekwondo, Brazilian jiu-jitsu, kung fu, and beyond—to submit their biographies. Tell us about your journey in martial arts, your teaching philosophy, and any significant contributions you've made to the field. Along with your biography.

Join Us in Celebrating Martial Arts The *International Martial Arts Instructors Guide 2025* is not just a book; it's a testament to the dedication, discipline, and hard work of martial artists around the globe. Don't miss this chance to be featured in this groundbreaking publication available exclusively online through *Amazon*. Be part of something extraordinary. Submit your biography today and help us showcase the vibrant and diverse world of martial arts! Your story is waiting to be told.

Free Submission: There's no cost to participate!

Please include: - *High-Quality Photos:* Submit images of yourself in uniform or Gi, showcasing your martial arts spirit and professionalism. -

Ensure we can reach you for any follow-up needed.

How to Submit Ready to make your mark? It's easy! Simply send your biographies and photos to us at artseastpublish@gmail.com. Remember, the deadline for submissions is approaching, so act fast!

SUBMIT

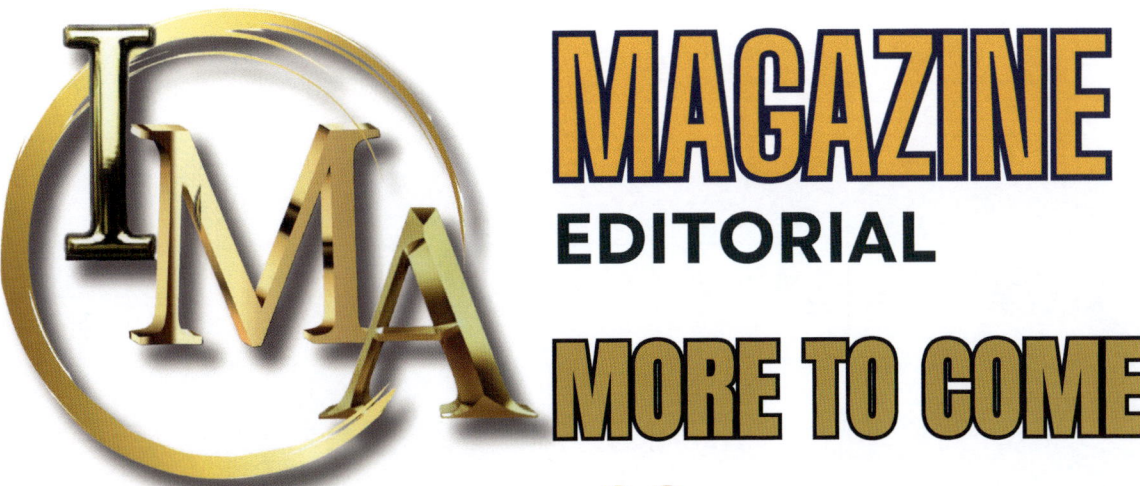

MAGAZINE
EDITORIAL
MORE TO COME

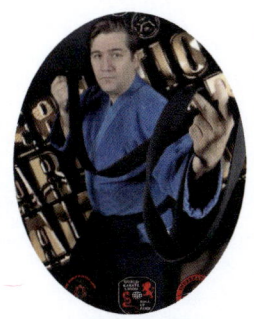

Here we are again, and even better than before, as we continue our journey forward with this month's exciting issue!

This edition is dedicated to celebrating the unsung heroes of the martial arts world, particularly focusing on the remarkable contributions of women

If you've been following our regular columns, you know that we often highlight female instructors and artists in Sumiko Nakano's monthly "Women Warriors" section.

However, this time, we've made a bold decision to dedicate the entire issue to female fighters, instructors, and martial artists who have often been undervalued and overlooked.

Their stories deserve to be told, and we are honored to showcase their incredible talents and achievements.

This issue features the legendary Queen of Martial Arts Cinema, Cynthia Rothrock, who graces our pages fresh off the success of her new hit film, **Black Creek**. Her insights into the film industry and martial arts journey are sure to inspire.

Additionally, we welcome back Michelle Manu, who shares her expertise in an engaging article on fighting skills that will empower our readers.

We also have an introspective piece from Gloria Hendry, famed as a Bond girl and star of the cult classic **Black Belt Jones**, reflecting on her unique experiences in the martial arts world.

Sumiko Nakano takes us on a deeper dive into the historical contributions of women in martial arts, shedding light on those who have paved the way for future generations. Our talented roster of notable instructors also returns with their regular contributions, enriching our magazine with diverse perspectives and we are thrilled to announce that our readership has already surpassed 190,000 views, and we continue to grow!

Your support fuels our passion for bringing you the best content in the martial arts community.

Looking ahead, we have an exciting lineup for future issues, including features on Mark Shuey, the cane master, Grandmaster Eric Lee, and action icon Michael Jai White, to name just a few. The journey of exploring martial arts continues, and we invite you to keep following us here at IMA Magazine.

May 2025 / Vol. 2 - No. 5

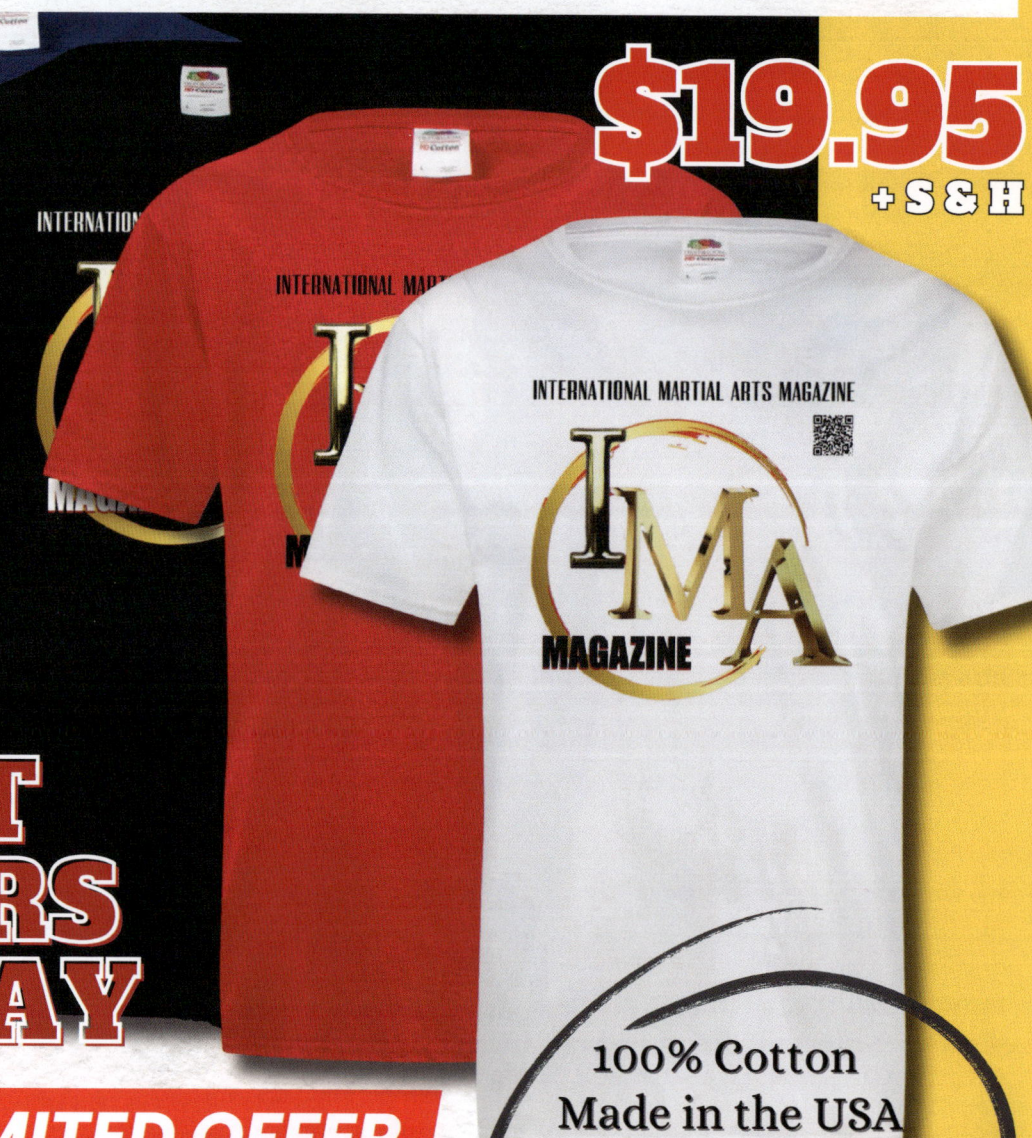

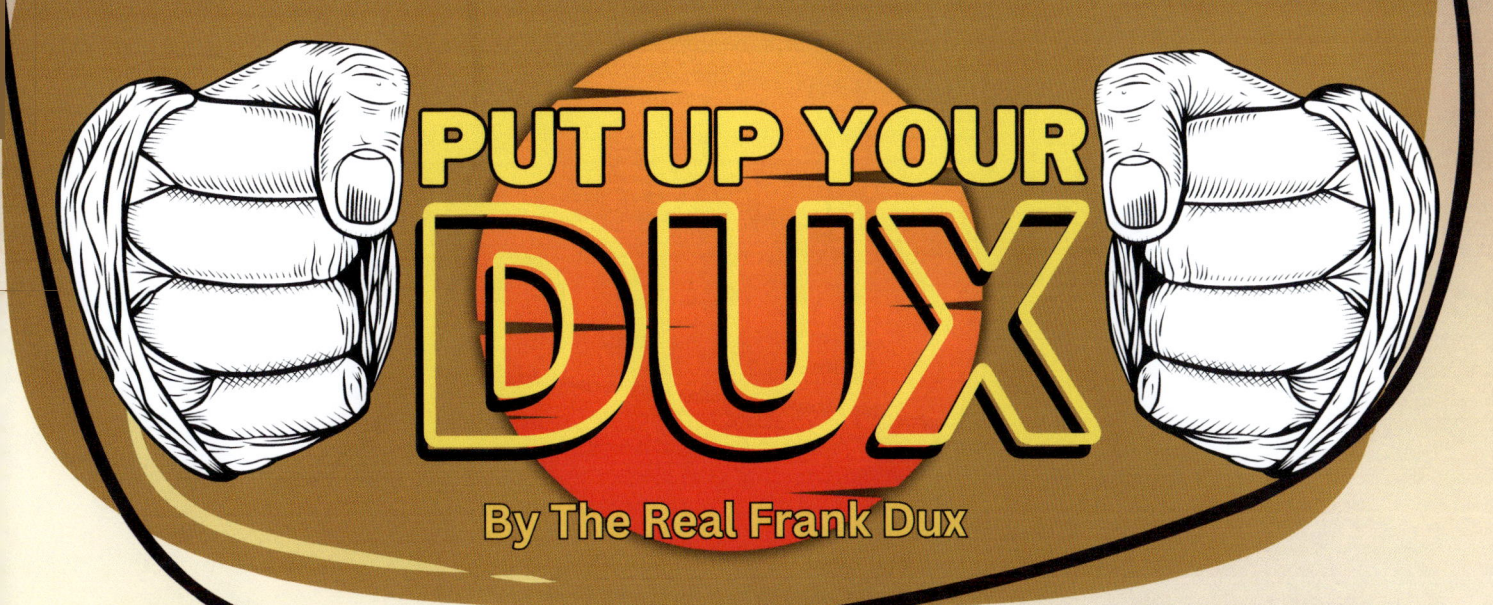

PUT UP YOUR DUX
By The Real Frank Dux

WOMEN IN MARTIAL ARTS

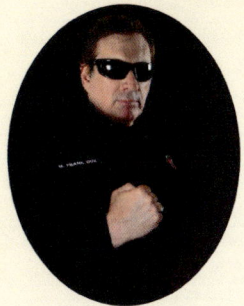

I began my journey into martial arts world in the mid 1960's, when societal attitudes regarding gender equality were just beginning to evolve.

Females in cinema and television suddenly went from being that damsel in distress needing to be saved to saving others using martial arts on popular TV shows and films, ergo Gloria Hendry, 007 Bond girl and Black belt Jones, Emma Peel from The Avengers and all the beautiful women in Man From Uncle, etc.

The era of Sport Karate and Judo was just coming into its own in the mid-1960's. That also provided new opportunities for women. This change coincided with the rise of movements advocating for women's rights, which, in turn, visibly sparked growing interest in martial arts among women.

One of the first signs of significant change came in the 1970s and 1980s, when martial arts organizations were actively promoting training and organizing tournaments for female practitioners.

The predominate male participants played a crucial role in fostering a supportive environment for women who wanted to engage in martial arts that had previously been considered predominantly restricted to male athletes.

The advent of women's tournaments was pivotal milestone in this evolution that gave women a platform to demonstrate their skills and compete at the highest levels.

The increasing visibility of female competitors helped shift public perception to the extent that female athletes went from not just being viewed as participants but valuable contributors to the martial arts community.

Women began to be represented in major competitions, including the Olympics, further solidifying their place in martial arts.

The inclusion of women in such high-profile events highlighted the physical prowess of female athletes.

It was partly responsible for societal shifts toward gender equality, leaving a lasting mark on the world.

The history of women in martial arts is not a recent phenomenon as critics of female teachers would have others believe. Women in martial arts spans centuries and transcends cultural boundaries.

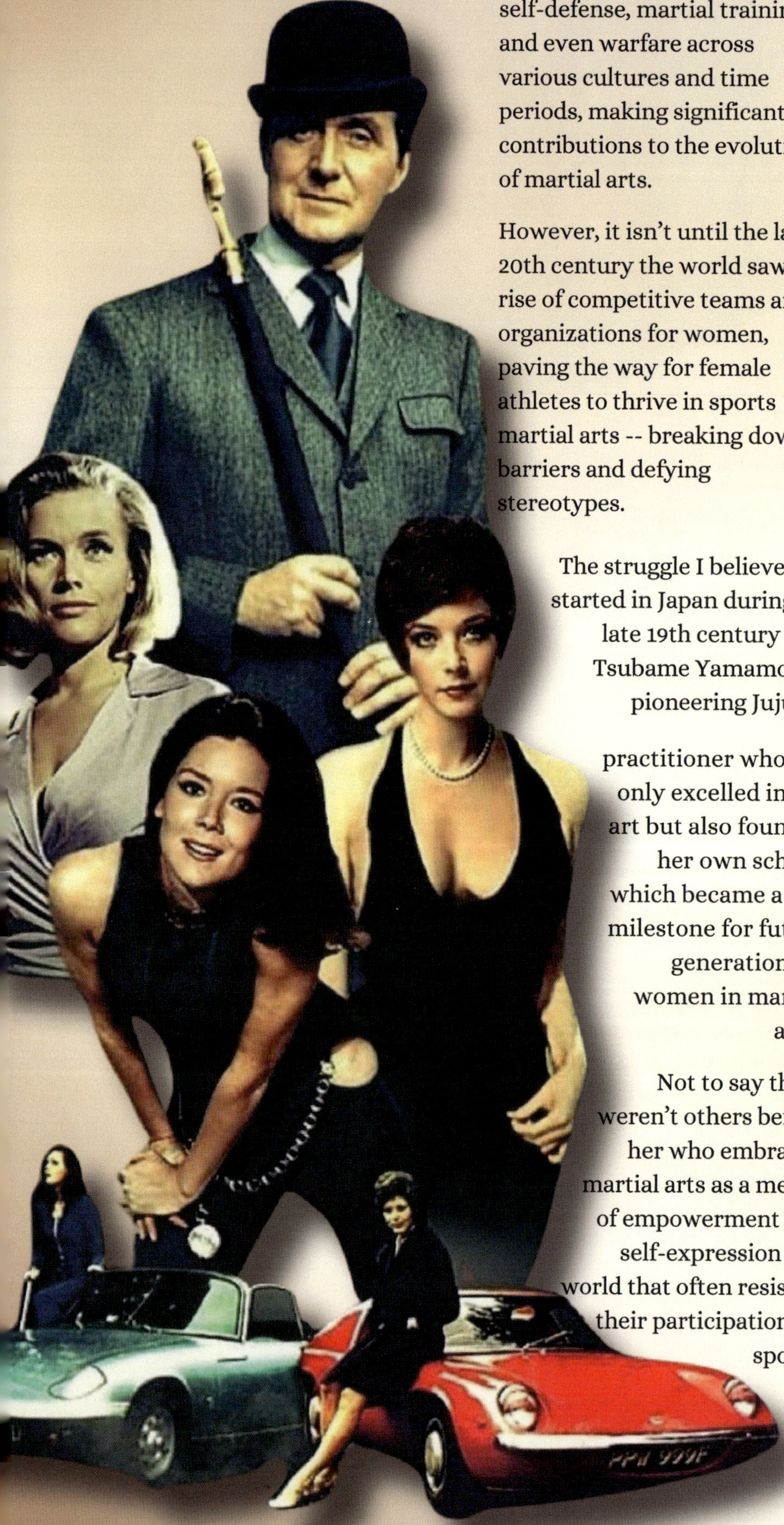

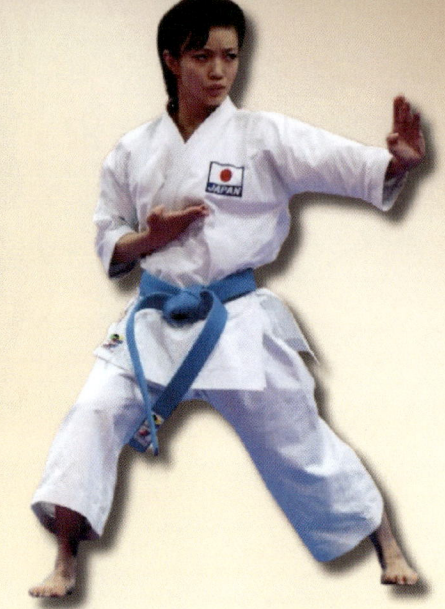

Women have long engaged in self-defense, martial training, and even warfare across various cultures and time periods, making significant contributions to the evolution of martial arts.

However, it isn't until the late 20th century the world saw the rise of competitive teams and organizations for women, paving the way for female athletes to thrive in sports martial arts -- breaking down barriers and defying stereotypes.

The struggle I believe first started in Japan during the late 19th century with Tsubame Yamamoto, a pioneering Jujutsu practitioner who not only excelled in the art but also founded her own school, which became a key milestone for future generations of women in martial arts.

Not to say there weren't others before her who embraced martial arts as a means of empowerment and self-expression in a world that often resisted their participation in sports.

Female martial artists have balanced the roles of practitioners and instructors while challenging ingrained stereotypes.

Despite the societal obstacles they faced, female martial artists laid the foundation for the rise of feminist ideals in the sports world -- advocating for equality and representation. Their legacy continues to resonate, underscoring the essential role women have played in martial arts history.

On a personal note, having seen actual combat I can confidently say there are some women operators trust and would pick to fight alongside over muscle headed bearded macho men full of bravado and that's about all they have going for them.

Gender doesn't determine victory, skill meeting opportunity with determination, this favors a desired outcome.

Frank Dux

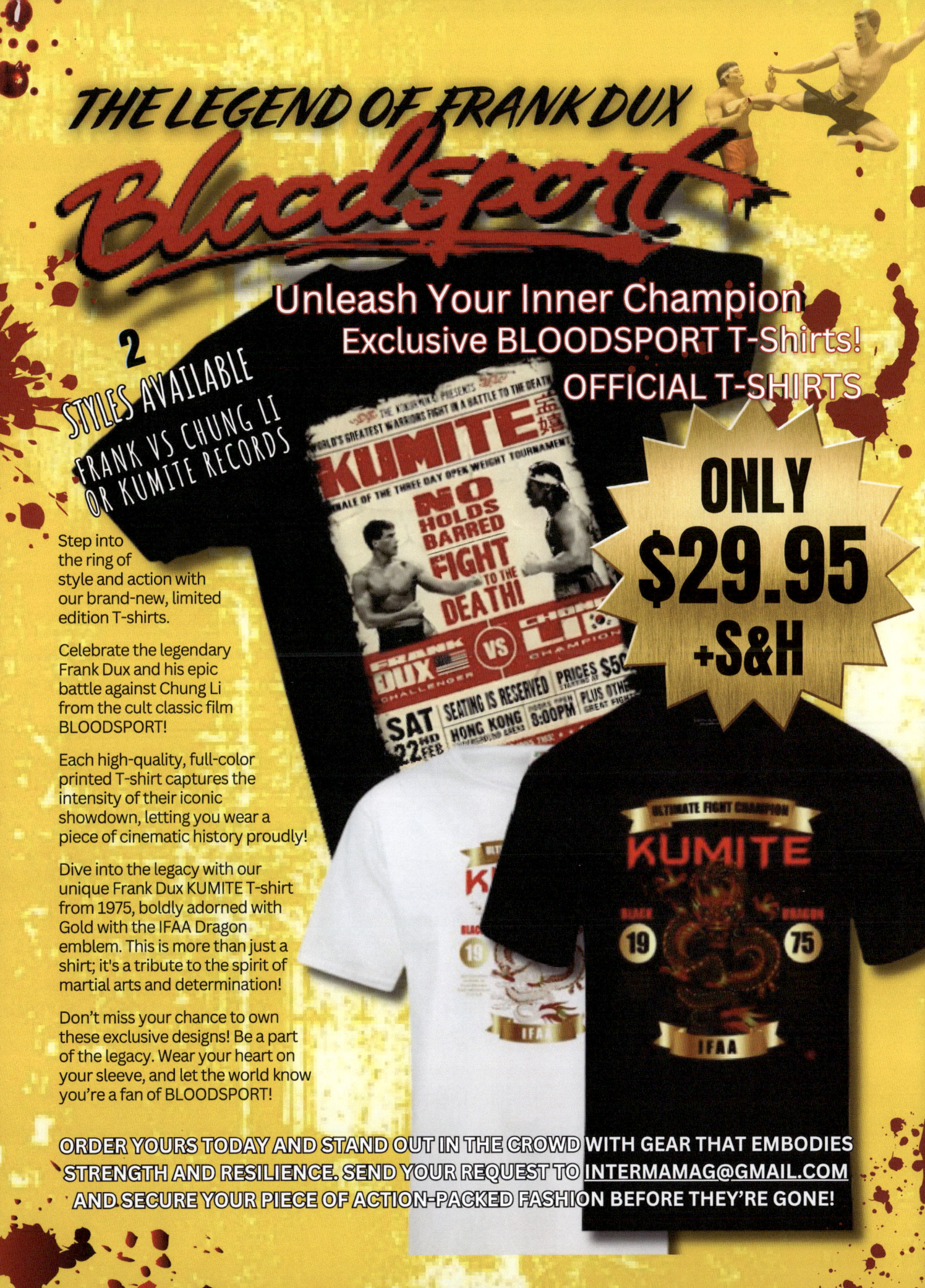

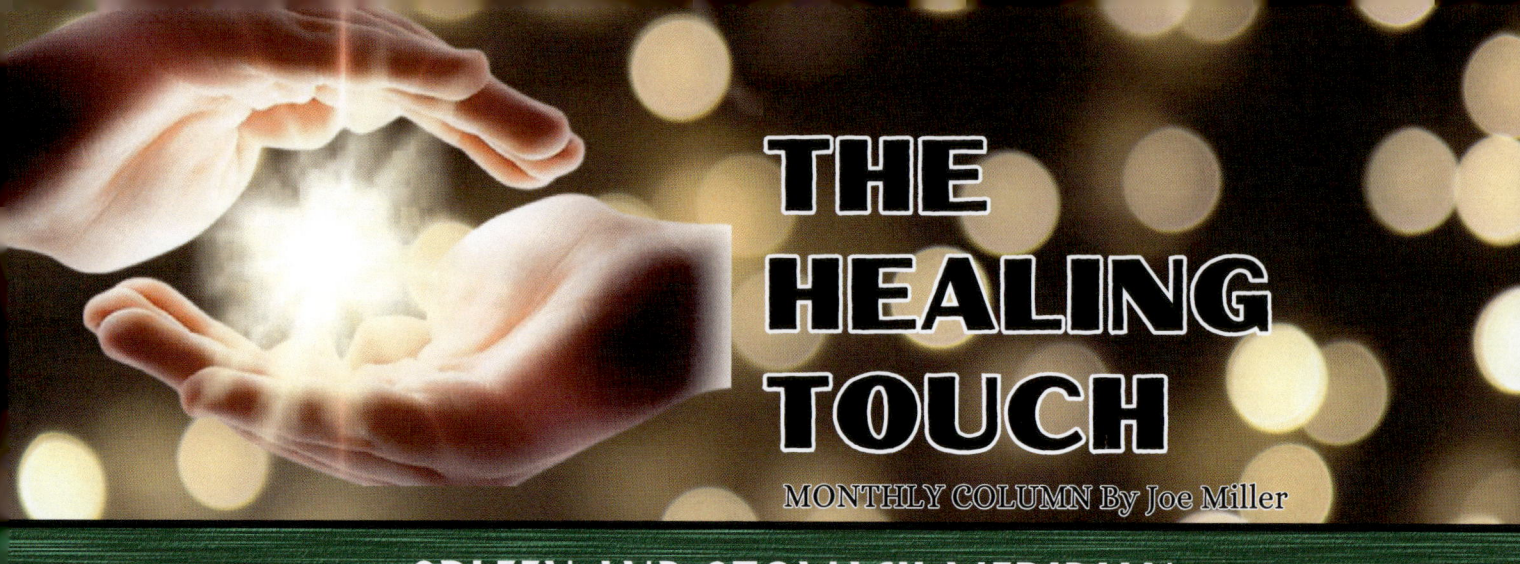

THE HEALING TOUCH

MONTHLY COLUMN By Joe Miller

SPLEEN AND STOMACH MERIDIAN

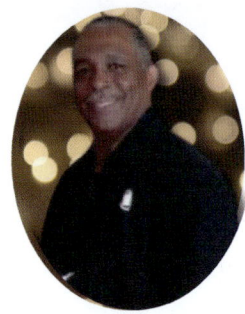

The spleen and stomach meridians are part of the traditional Chinese medicine (TCM) system, which views the body as a network of energy pathways called meridians. Each meridian is associated with specific organs and functions.

- The spleen meridian is responsible for transforming and transporting nutrients throughout the body. It plays a crucial role in digestion, absorption, and the production of qi (vital energy) and blood.
- It is believed to help regulate the body's fluids and is associated with the muscles and flesh.

- Emotionally, the spleen is linked to worry and overthinking.

And it is paired with the Stomach Meridian: which is a Yo meridian in Japanese terminology and Yang in TCM.

- The stomach meridian works closely with the spleen meridian and is primarily responsible for the initial stages of digestion.

- It governs the breakdown of food and the extraction of nutrients, which are then transformed and transported by the spleen.

- The stomach meridian is associated with the body's ability to nourish itself and maintain energy levels.

The spleen Meridian is also known as the triple heater of the stomach organs.

The spleen and stomach meridians work together to ensure proper digestion and energy distribution.

In TCM and Japanese Shiatsu, maintaining balance and harmony between these meridians is crucial for overall health and well-being.

SPLEEN ANATOMY

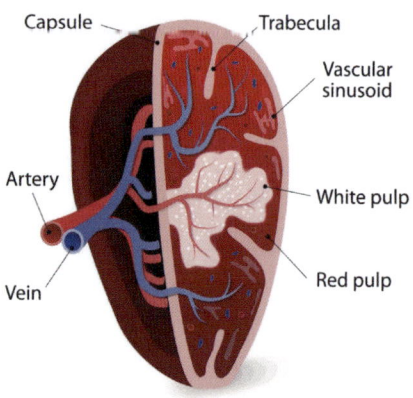

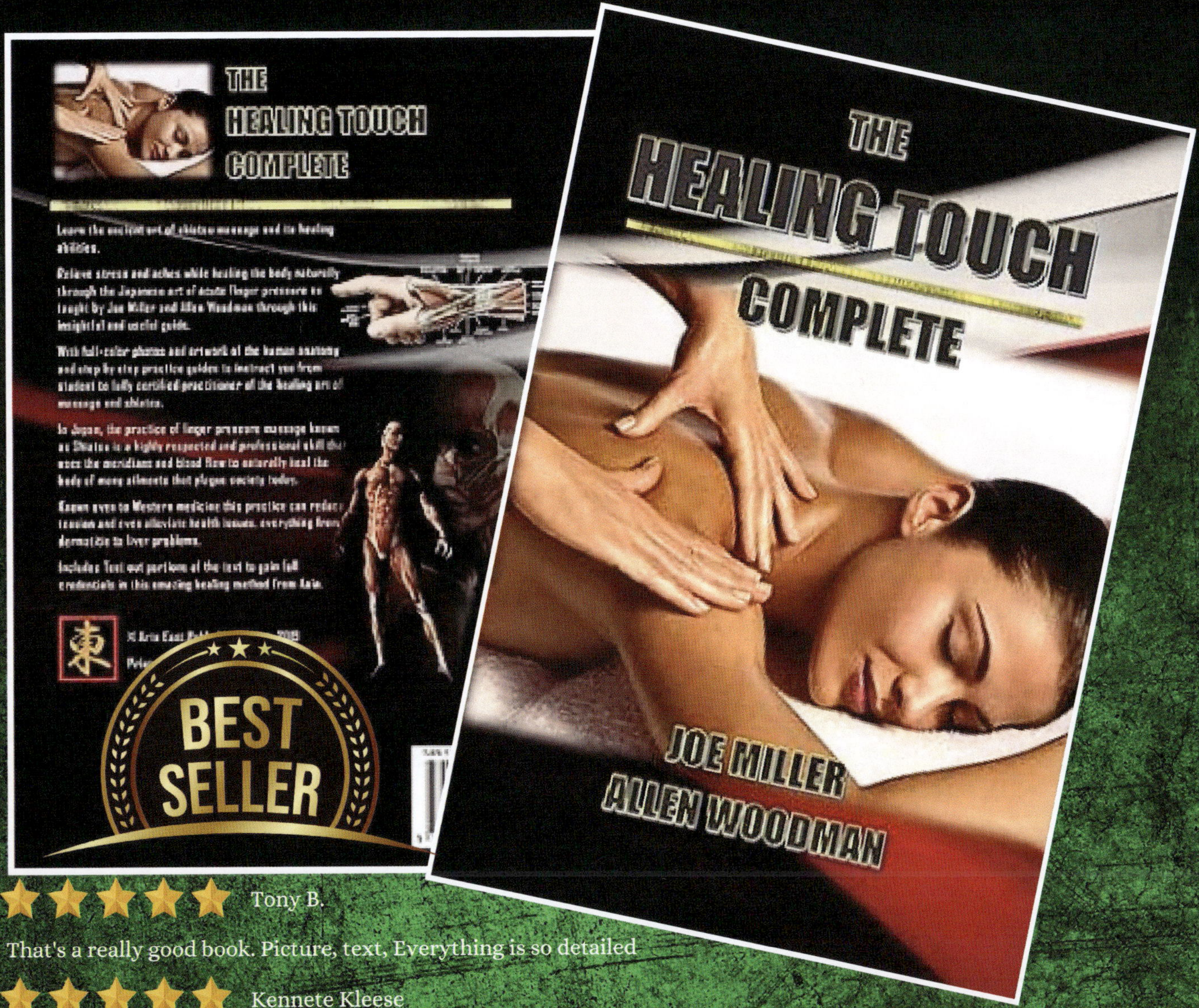

★★★★★ Tony B.
That's a really good book. Picture, text, Everything is so detailed

★★★★★ Kennete Kleese
The book is understandable whether you are a beginner or advance student or professional of any style of massage

★★★★★ Barry Southam
Great text to add to your library.

Learn the ancient art of shiatsu massage and its healing abilities. Relieve stress and aches while healing the body naturally through the Japanese art of acute finger pressure through this insightful and useful guide. With full-color photos and artwork of the human anatomy and step by step practice guides to instruct you from student to fully certified practitioner. In Japan, the practice of finger pressure massage known as Shiatsu is a highly respected, professional skill that uses the meridians and blood flow to naturally heal the body. Shiatsu can reduce tension and even alleviate health issues. Includes Test out portions of the text to gain full credentials in this amazing healing method from Asia.

- Language : English
- Paperback : 299 pages
- Dimensions : 7 x 0.71 x 10 inches

LIMITED
$69.95
FREE DELIVERY

QUALITY GUARANTEED

AVAILABLE ON AMAZON.COM

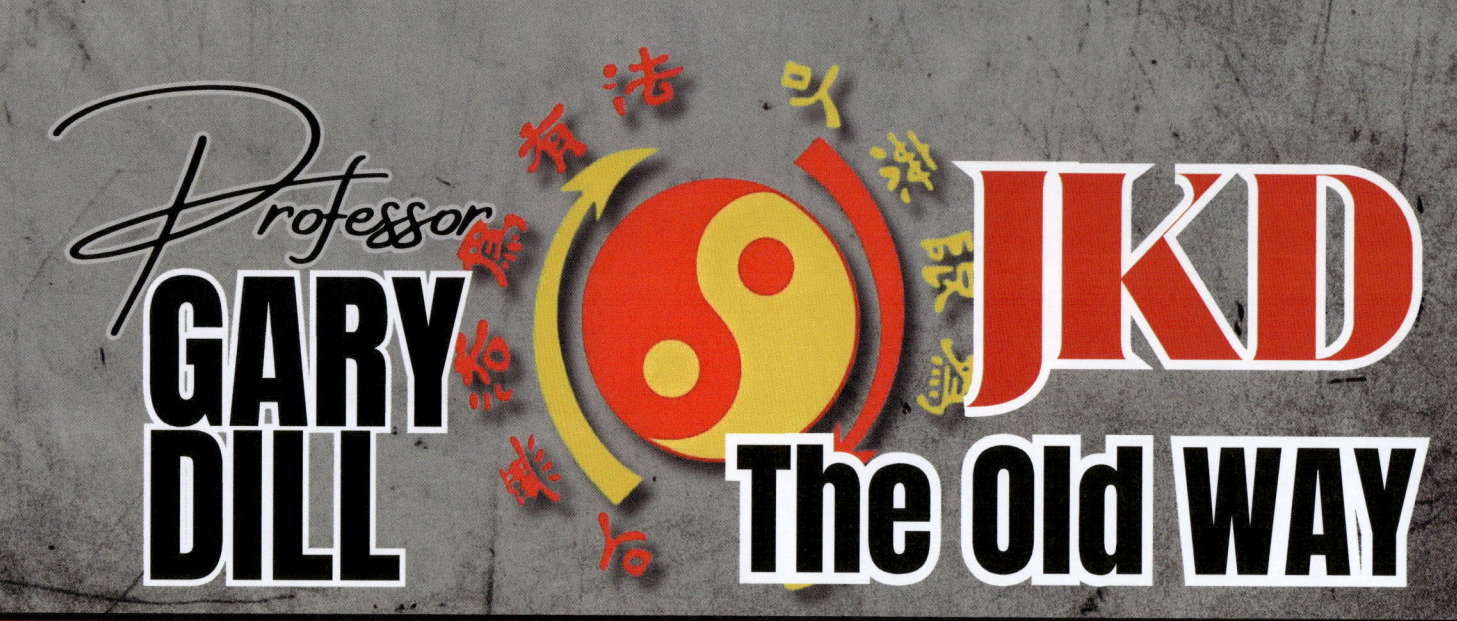

Professor GARY DILL
JKD The Old WAY

THE JEET KUNE DO SOCIETY

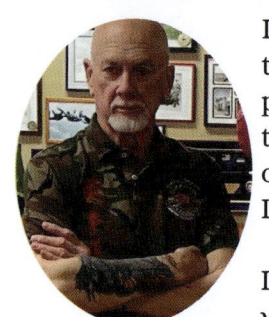

I can presume that most JKD practitioners today never heard of the Jeet Kune Do Society.

In 1986 the Society was formed as the first attempt in unifying the different factions of JKD for the purpose of universal certification, continuity of training, and developing a brotherhood among the membership. The Society had an impressive leadership roster.

Honorary Executives were Linda Lee and Taky Kimura. Dan Inosanto was the Executive Director with Richard Bustillo being the Chairman of the Board. The Board of Directors was comprised of only original students.

The Society started in 1986 was when Bustillo sent 'letters to the Editor" to the major martial arts magazines searching for students who actually trained in either Seattle, Oakland, or LA Chinatown, who would be interested in joining the newly formed JKD Society.

The applicant was required to send in a resume', photo, any documentation and $25 registration fee. In 1971-72 I was one of the original students at the Oakland school taught by James Yimm Lee.

Bruce was still in charge of the training and curriculum even though he was in Hong Kong making movies.

I wanted to be a part of a national JKD organization and submitted my application with several documents verifying my authenticity.

I immediately received a reply letter from Bustillo advising me that my application was being vetted.

In 1985, before I even knew anything about the JKD Society, I had met Dan Inosanto at one of his seminars in Dallas. We hit it off and he invited me up to his room and we discussed James Lee and the Oakland JKD curriculum. He referred to James as being his "big brother" in JKD.

After about an hour Master Chai came into the hotel room and we ended up having a group conversation for the next two hours.

I received a second letter from Bustillo. It stated that all of my credentials were authentic and that Dan had also personally vouched for me.

Bustillo immediately appointed me to be on the Society Board of Directors representing Oakland and the deceased James Lee.

This was a great honor and privilege for me.

There was membership certificates issued as well as a monthly newsletter, the Jeet Kune Do Journal.

The headquarters was located at the IMB Academy in Torrance, California, which at that time was a very large facility.

In late 1986, one of my senior Kempo instructors, David Hinkle, and I flew to LA for my first Society meeting. This was a very important meeting. We were finalizing the final draft of the new Society constitution and by-laws.

When we arrived, everyone was dressed in casual clothes. Hinkle and I were wearing suits and ties. Bustillo asked why we were so formal, and I replied that Master Hinkle has an MBA and was a director of a state agency in Oklahoma, and that I was a former federal agent and Chief of Police.

This was our usual attire for formal meetings. Bustillo said that we were in California now.

Everyone laughed and we settled down to work.

We went over all of the aspects of the constitution and by-laws making numerous changes and finally it was completed.

That part of the meeting was over and now for more new business. Bustillo said that the Society was approved by Linda Lee as the official voice for Bruce Lee (since he had been dead for over 13 years) and the Society could act and make JKD decisions in his name. He then added that a strong foundation of authentic JKD instructors were needed to be in place to help educated and teach new members. (Remember, Bruce only named three instructors, Taky, James, and Dan.)

Consequently Richard, as the Chairman of the Board, announced that all members of the Board of Directors were now officially recognized as "Full Instructors" of JKD. James gave me written permission in December 1972 (just before he died) to "share" my knowledge of JKD to my students in Oklahoma, but he could not make me a formal instructor for only Bruce could make instructors.

Richard told me after the meeting that was standard policy during that time, whereas the "big three" could give their senior students permission to "share" JKD.

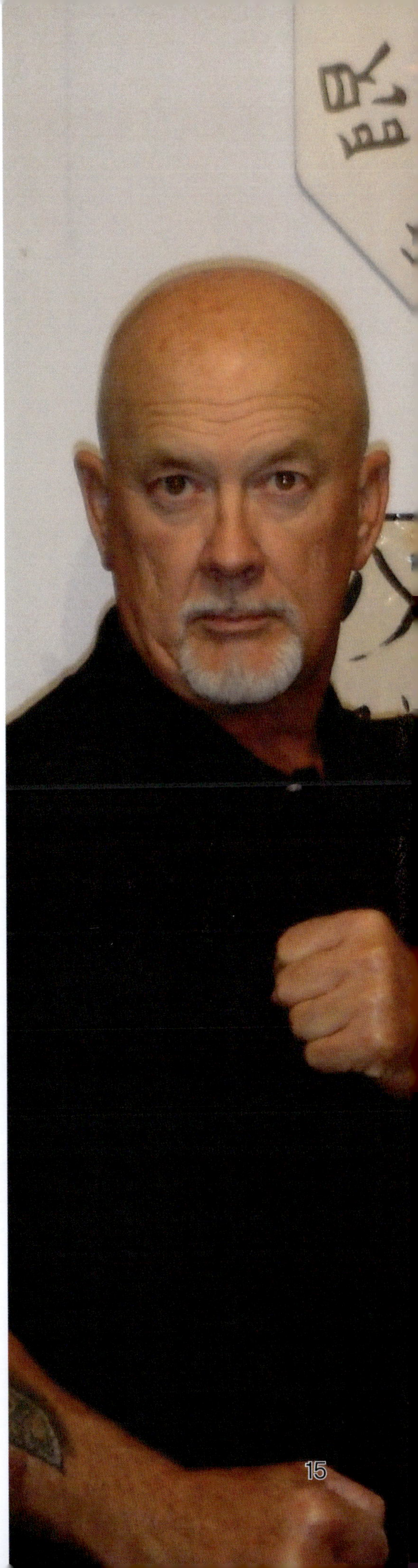

May 2025 / Vol. 2 - No. 5

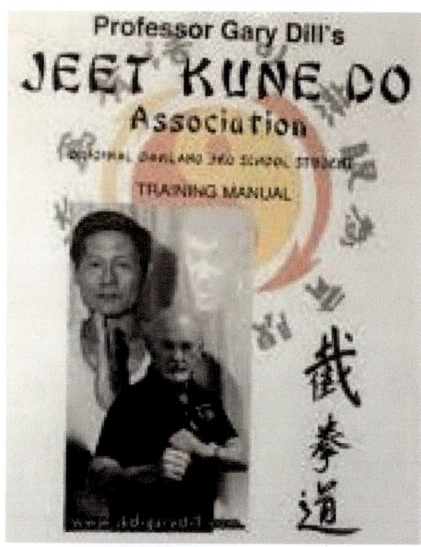

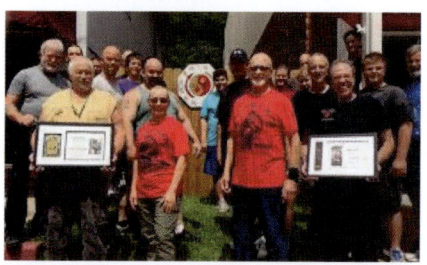

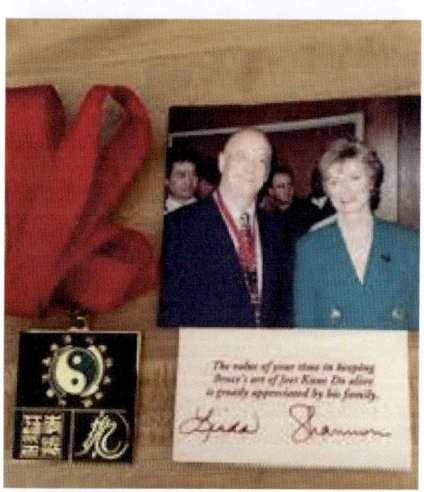

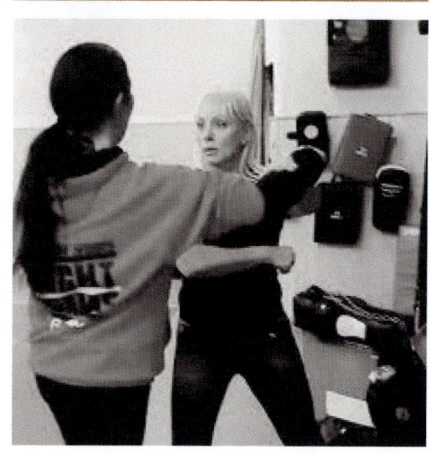

Richard added that I'm fortunate to have this permission to share JKD in writing because everyone else only had verbal permission. Consequently, I was certified/recognized by the JKD Society as a "Full Instructor" of Jeet Kune Do.

Richard said that the Society sent in the JKD Logo (yin/yang with arrows and calligraphy surrounding it) as well as the name "Jeet Kune Do" to the US Patent Office to be officially designated as registered trademarks officially owned by the JKD Society. But since they had been used for 13 years by the public, they were considered now as "Public Domain" and can be used by anyone, with no one having ownership of the logo or name.

Over the next year or two of operation, the JKD Society never did develop momentum and got very few JKD practitioners to participate. It was like trying to herd a group of alley cats.

The Society, as it was originally formed, was disbanded, reorganized and absorbed within the IMB academy and the members of the Board were now only LA Chinatown students.

The JKD Society eventually dissolved and disappeared. But I expected this outcome. As a group, the Society strongly advocated the JKD Concepts (Kali, Escrima, Muay Thai, etc) whereas I taught the original, pre-1973 JKD curriculum as taught in the Oakland "Fighting School." So, in actuality, it became the JKD / IMB Concepts Society. I left the Society before its demise because of conflict of JKD philosophy. I think Jerry Poteet left before me and he was also an advocate of the pre-73 JKD.

In 1991, I formed the Jeet Kune Do Association which is based out of Oklahoma and have numerous affiliate schools and instructors across the US and internationally.

We specialize in the teaching and certification in the Oakland based original Jeet Kune Do (Wing Chun, Boxing, and Fencing.) I am frequently teaching seminars and private classes sharing the fighting skills and techniques of the Oakland JKD as it was developed by Bruce Lee.

Today, after 34 years, the JKD Association is the largest and longest standing JKD training organization in the world.

Professor Gary Dill

SEMINARS
NOW AVAILABLE

LEARN FROM THE SOURCE

- Learn the authentic JKD developed by Bruce Lee
- Taught by Gary Dill,
- 1st generation Oakland JKD student.
- Learn JKD punching, striking, low kicks, entering techniques, counter against blocks, block & counters
- Develop speed & proper techniques.

Contact Prof. Gary Dill directly at pdilljkd@aol.com.
Website: www.jkd-garydill.com
Contact 1 (918) 327-6895

Sifu George Hajnasr's

JEET KUNE DO
THE SYSTEM WITHOUT A SYSTEM

AVAILABLE NOW

$29.95

Jeet Kune Do A System Without a System is one of the best books ever written on the complete system that was pioneered by the late great Bruce Lee. George Hajnasr has put together the full course and understanding principles that are the make up of the complete system. Everything from Warm Up exercises to self defense techniques ranging from beginner to advanced. You will find it all in this one large manual of the Complete system of Jeet Kune DO A System Without a System.

502 pages
Language English
Publication February 3, 2014
Dimensions 8.5 x 1.01 x 11.02

BEST PRICE

AVAILABLE ON AMAZON.COM

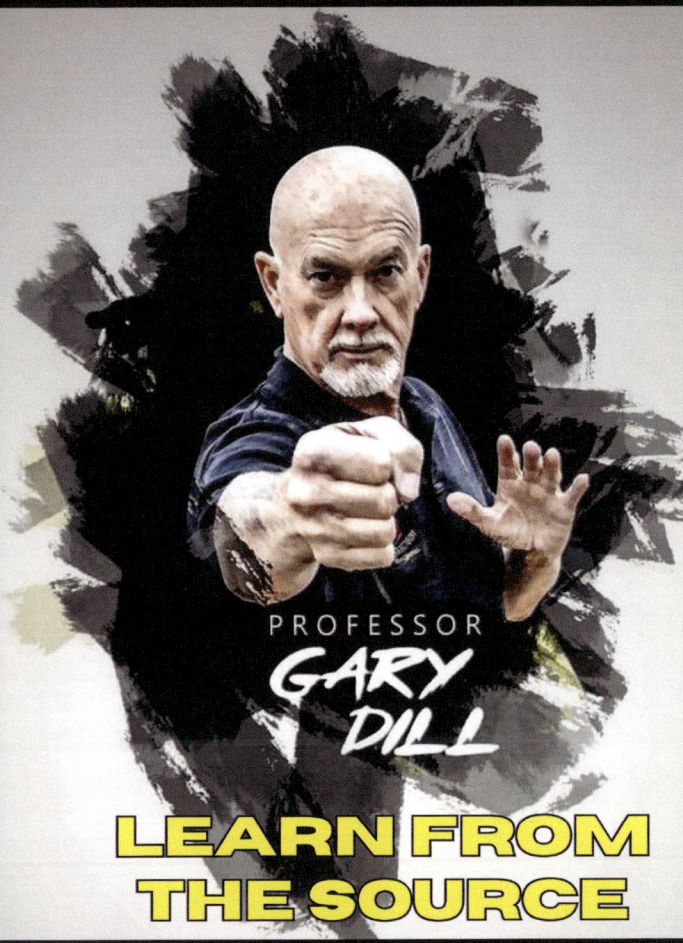

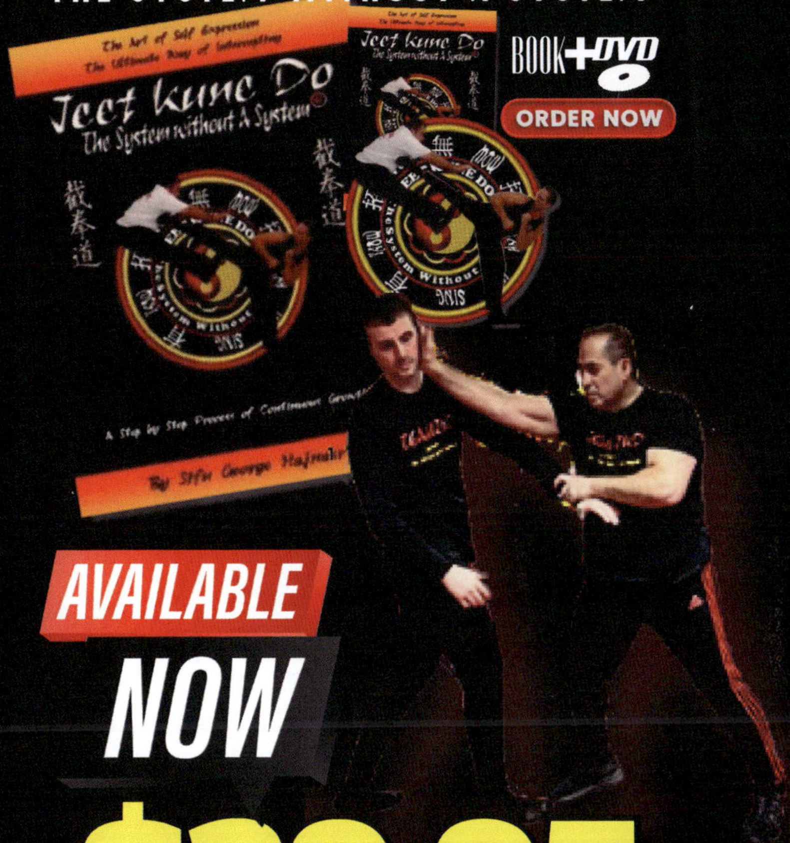

MARTIAL SCIENCE

A Comprehensive Exploration of Biomechanics, Anatomy, and Strategic Application

MARTIAL SCIENCE

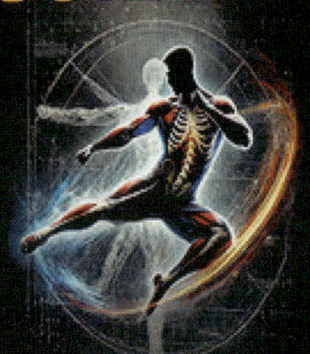

ORDER NOW — AVAILABLE ON AMAZON.COM

WHO SHOULD READ THIS BOOK

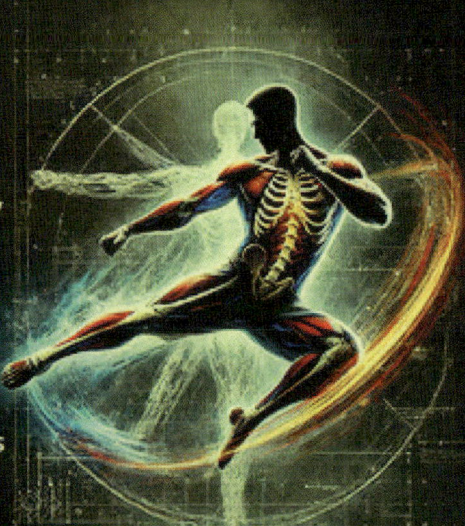

MARTIAL ARTISTS & FIGHTERS
- Master biomechanics for explosive power & efficiency
- Enhance strikes, grappling, and movement strategy

COACHES & TRAINERS
- Teach science-backed techniques for better results
- Prevent injuries & optimize performance

SELF-DEFENSE ENTHUSIASTS
- Learn efficient, real-world combat applications
- Understand leverage, timing, and adaptability

TRAIN SMARTER, MOVE FASTER, STRIKE HARDER!
- Discover the science behind every move and take your skills to the next level!

WOMEN WARRIORS
GLORIA HENDRY
BUNNY TO BOND GIRL

By Sumiko Nakano
& Allen Woodman

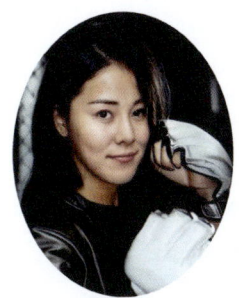

You think you know what a Bond girl is supposed to be—glamorous, fragile, expendable.

Then Gloria Hendry walks onto the screen, and suddenly the rules don't apply. She's Rosie Carver in Live and Let Die—armed, defiant, dangerous.

The first Black woman to ever share a bed with James Bond, and far more than just a footnote in film history. But the truth is, Gloria was never just a Bond girl. She was raised in Newark, New Jersey—tough, athletic, and unafraid to go head-to-head with the world. She didn't come from money or legacy.

She came from motion. Track. Gymnastics. Street smarts and muscle memory. From an early age, she was fighting—fighting systems, fighting perceptions, and sometimes, just straight-up fighting. She turned heads in fashion and threw punches in film.

"I never thought of being an actress originally,"

She tells me, her voice low but unwavering.

"I'd go to the theater and sit as close to the front screen as possible. It pulled me in, but I didn't imagine I could belong on the screen."

She didn't just belong—she owned it.

Gloria Hendry was born in Jacksonville, Florida. That same fire followed her north to Newark, where she pushed into modeling with poise, grit, and a glare that told people not to waste her time.

From modeling, she jumped into acting—accidentally, really.

May 2025 / Vol. 2 - No. 5

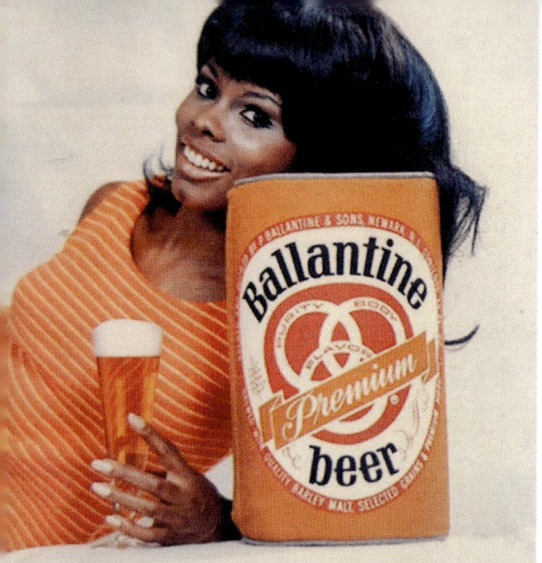

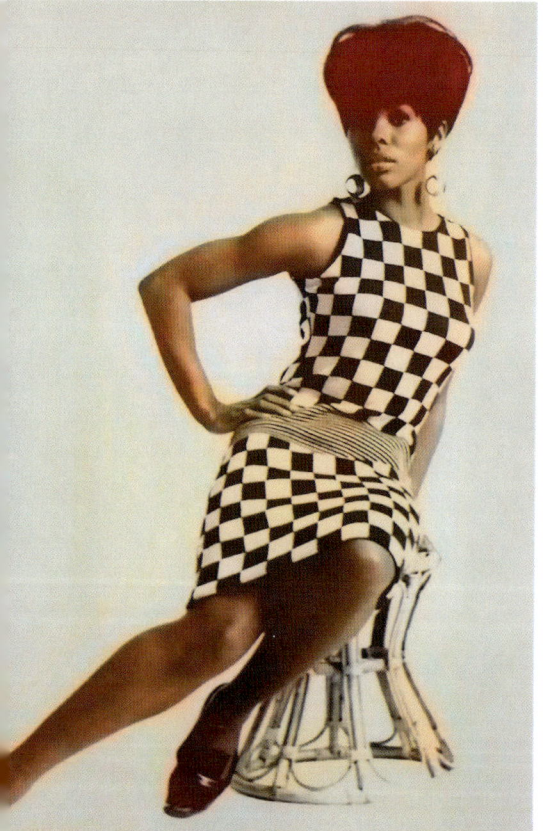

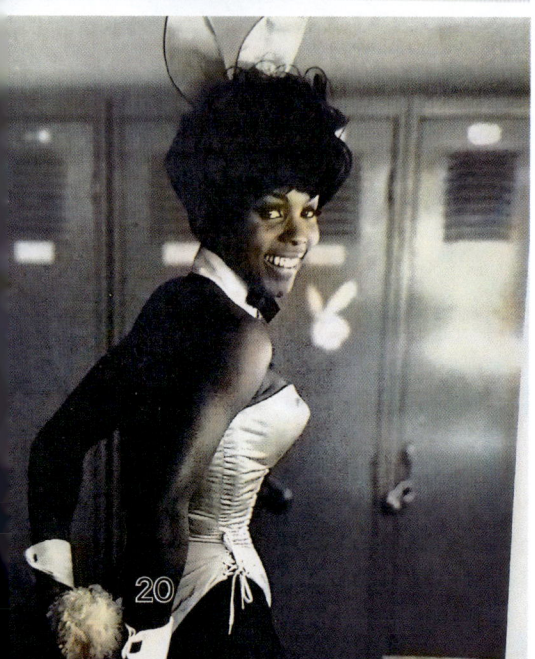

She wasn't chasing fame. But it kept showing up.

When she landed Live and Let Die in 1973, it was historic. Not that anyone told her that.

"I didn't really think about being anyone special. It just happened as I did it,"

She says.

"I struggled with the fact that I never walked around trying to be anything other than what I am."

Rosie Carver wasn't just a love interest. She was a CIA agent, someone with her own agenda, her own weapons. And for Black audiences—especially women—she was something they hadn't seen before: a Black woman on screen who wasn't comic relief, wasn't cleaning up after someone, wasn't background.

She was central. She was complex. And she was beautiful without being anyone's fantasy.

Gloria didn't play Rosie as decoration. She played her as a woman who could hold her own—and maybe couldn't be trusted. It was a revelation.

I could be just as good as any man,"

She says simply. That was her quiet rebellion.

She never begged to be accepted. She was the standard. People just hadn't caught up yet.

Gloria wasn't just turning heads in spy thrillers. She was flipping bodies in action films before most studios thought Black women could even throw a punch on screen.

"I was one of the first Black women to do martial arts in film,"

she tells me, correcting a note from earlier.

"Not the first—but one of the first, and that was before Pam Grier came on screen."

It was *Black Belt Jones* that cemented her as more than just a trailblazer—it made her dangerous.

Paired with Jim Kelly, she played Sydney, a fierce, stylish fighter who could deliver a side kick and a punchline without blinking. Gloria didn't just hold her own—she stole scenes with raw physical confidence.

From modeling, she jumped into acting—accidentally, really. She wasn't chasing fame. But it kept showing up.

When she landed Live and Let Die in 1973, it was historic. Not that anyone told her that.

May 2025 / Vol. 2 - No. 5

"I didn't really think about being anyone special. It just happened as I did it,"

She says.

"I struggled with the fact that I never walked around trying to be anything other than what I am."

Rosie Carver wasn't just a love interest. She was a CIA agent, someone with her own agenda, her own weapons.

For Black audiences—especially women—she was something they hadn't seen before: a Black woman on screen who wasn't comic relief, wasn't cleaning up after someone, wasn't background.

She was central. She was complex. And she was beautiful without being anyone's fantasy.

Gloria didn't play Rosie as decoration. She played her as a woman who could hold her own—and maybe couldn't be trusted.

It was a revelation.

"I could be just as good as any man,"

She says simply.

That was her quiet rebellion. She never begged to be accepted. She was the standard.

People just hadn't caught up yet.

Gloria wasn't just turning heads in spy thrillers.

She was flipping bodies in action films before most studios thought Black women could even throw a punch on screen.

"I was one of the first Black women to do martial arts in film,"

She tells me, correcting a note from earlier.

"Not the first—but one of the first, and that was before Pam Grier came on screen."

It was Black Belt Jones that cemented her as more than just a trailblazer—it made her dangerous.

Paired with the incomparable Jim Kelly, she played Sydney, a fierce, stylish fighter who could deliver a side kick and a punchline without blinking.

Gloria didn't just hold her own—she stole scenes with raw physical confidence.

"It was a true honor".

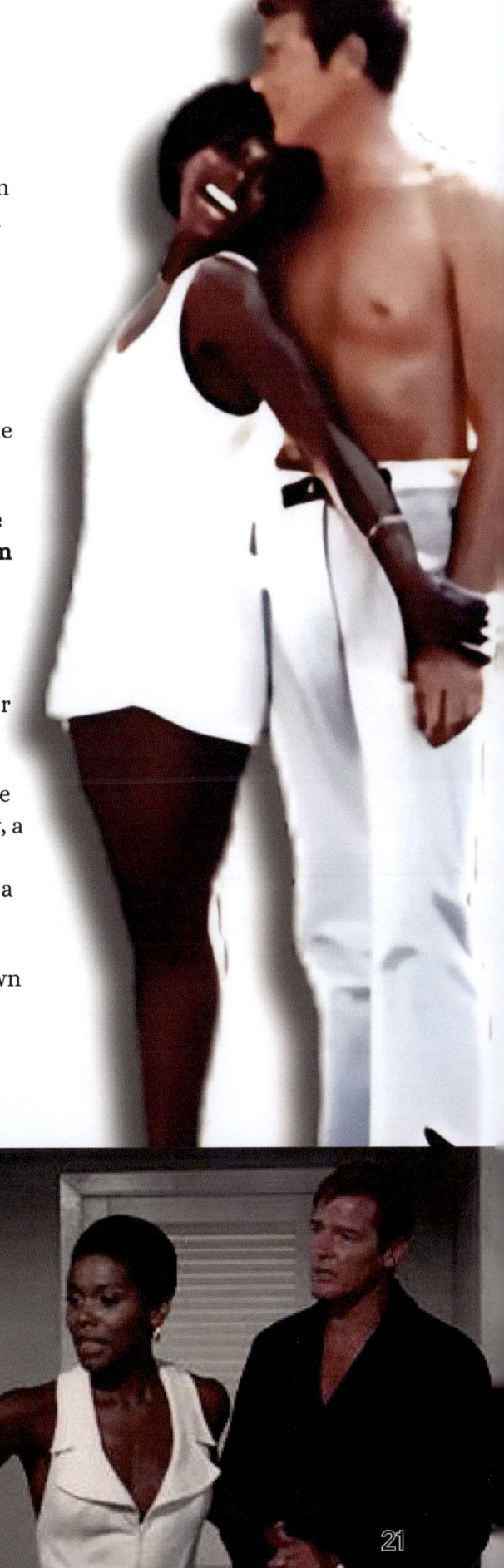

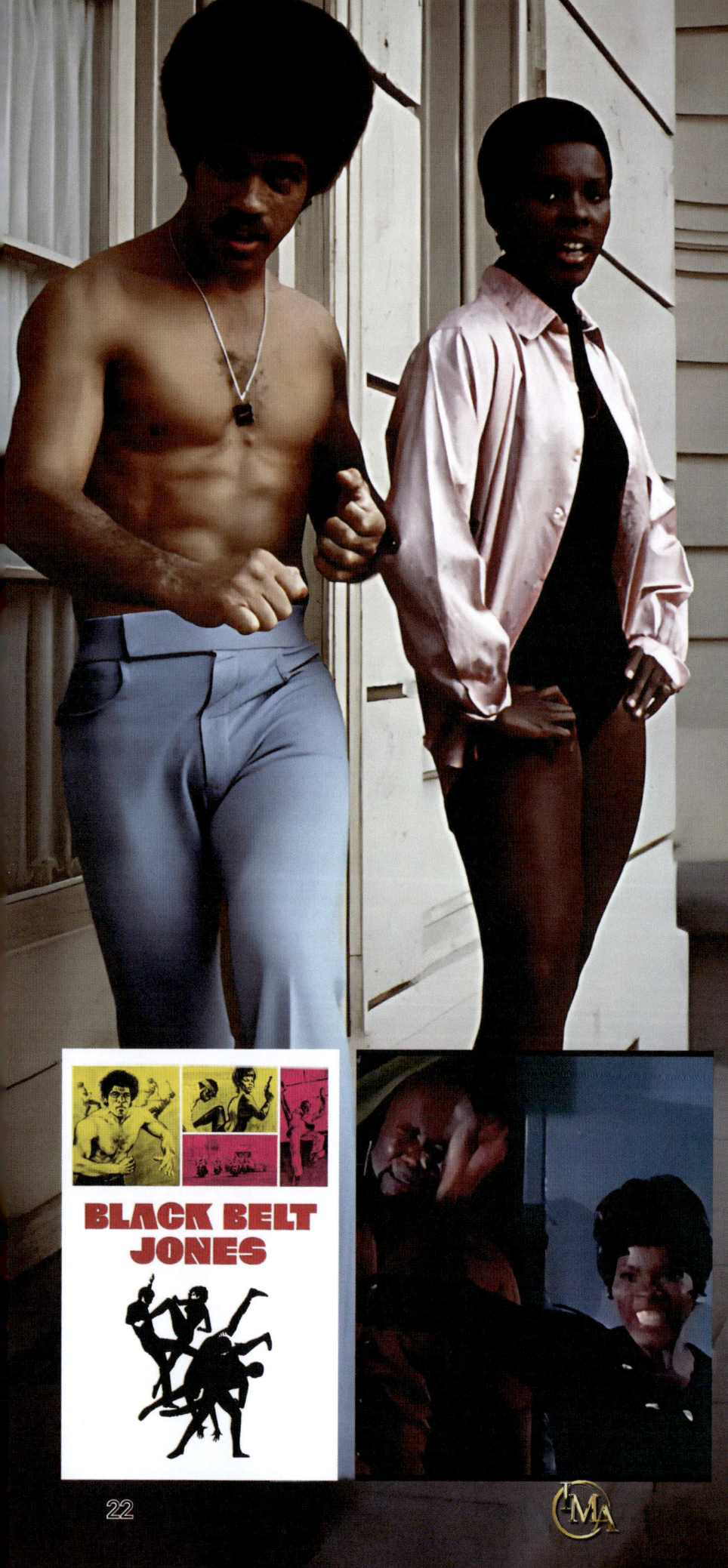

She says now, reflecting on her place in film history.

What's often overlooked is that Gloria wasn't some trained stunt double hiding behind edits.

She was athletic. She was capable. She knew how to move. She brought street-born agility into roles written with a flat male gaze—and blew those roles wide open.

She didn't just play strong women. She was one.

"I didn't want to be a secretary. Or a submissive role. I could do more than that."

And she did.

During the rise of the blaxploitation era—a time when Black actors were finally taking lead roles but still boxed into stereotypes—Gloria pushed through.

She starred in Black Caesar, Hell Up in Harlem, and Savage Sisters. These weren't prestige films. They weren't polished or subtle. But they gave Black actors something Hollywood hadn't: the front of the frame.

Gloria didn't waste the opportunity. She doesn't romanticize it. She knows the limitations.

"The most challenging thing was just getting into the business,"

she tells me.

May 2025 / Vol. 2 - No. 5

"It was a male-dominated industry."

What she doesn't say—but what you feel—is that she carved out space where none was given. Not because it was easy. But because she refused to settle.

These roles may not have come with Oscars. But they came with impact. For a generation of women who saw Gloria on screen—gun in hand, voice strong, body in motion—it was enough to change what they thought was possible.

What Gloria Hendry faced behind the scenes didn't always match the strength she projected on screen. Because while she played women who kicked down doors, the real battles were quieter—and much harder to win.

"As a woman of color, I take it as an affront, because I've always worked within the legal business as a legal secretary."

That tension—between who she was, who she portrayed, and how she was seen—was constant.

Gloria didn't have the luxury of pretending. The film industry wanted her to fit a mold. She refused. Even when it cost her.

She didn't ask to be a symbol. But she became one anyway.

"I never walked around trying to be anything other than what I am," she tells me. There's no self-pity in her voice, just clarity. That's who Gloria Hendry is: someone who didn't flinch when the door slammed, just kicked harder the next

Still, there were allies. People who saw her—not just the look or the attitude, but the work ethic underneath. She may have stood her ground alone more often than not, but she built her reputation on it. Even when the roles didn't come easy, even when the industry tried to typecast her or fade her out, Gloria found ways to keep going.

She started her own repertory theater company—a bold move then, still rare now.

"It still goes today,"

She says, with pride. It's the kind of legacy that doesn't make headlines, but changes lives.

Ask her what kind of role she'd play now, and she doesn't hesitate:

"Anything action or spy film. Anything that creates character. President of the United States would be a great role."

You believe her. Not just because she says it with conviction, but because she's earned it.

Because this business—this world—will try to convince you you're disposable if you don't fit the frame. Gloria never fit the frame. So she built her own.

Her message to women today is direct, and it hits like a final act monologue. Not written by a screenwriter. Lived.

"Women as a whole—love yourself the most. You are number one. The most important person. You can do anything you want to do. You never need anyone to tell you what you are or who you are. Strive to do better. Life is a big adventure. Go and adventure."

That's not a quote—it's a mission statement. It's what she would have told her younger self, standing on that set in 1973, being handed a role no one thought she deserved but one she made iconic. It's what she tells the young women now—especially those of color—walking into auditions, boardrooms, or battlefields stacked against them.

This isn't just motivation. It's strategy. Gloria Hendry doesn't preach dreams—she preaches action. Self-definition.

Adventure with armor.

Sumiko Nakano
Allen Woodman

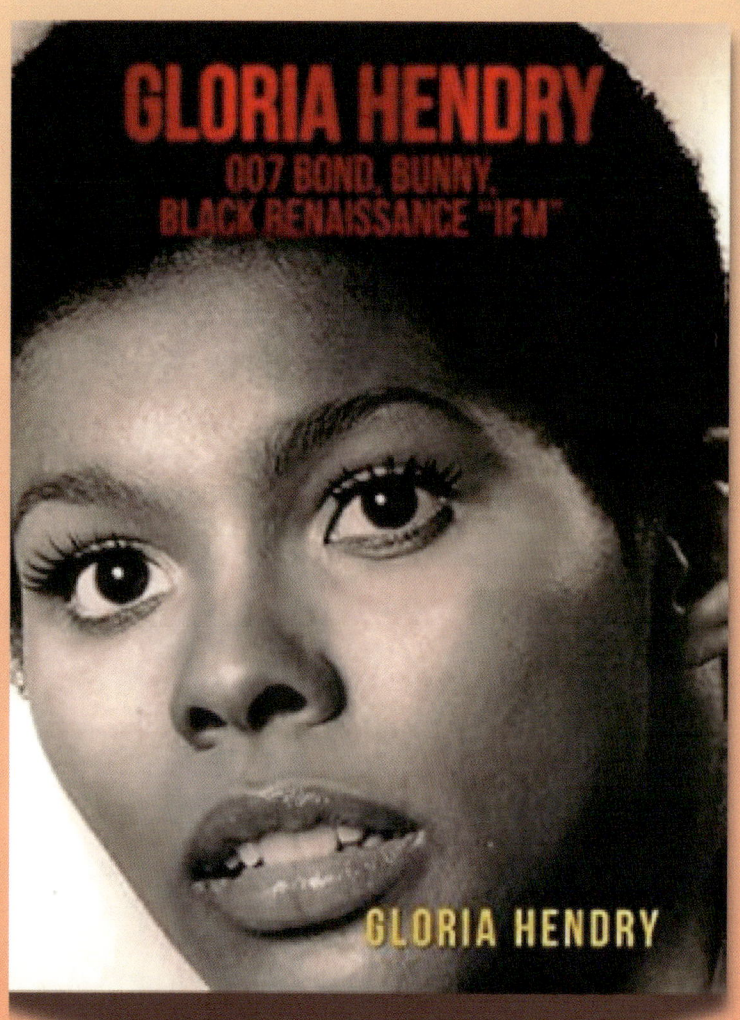

★★★★★

Powerful life story from a fabulous trail-blazer

Gloria Hendry is everything. Her life story is cinematic and inspiring, full of knock down drag out action and triumphant rising above. Before she became the first woman of color to be cast as a James Bond love interest, she worked for the NAACP, litigating cases during the Civil Rights Era. The journey from there to Playboy bunny to Bond girl is intense, and she talks about it all with such a beautifully irrepressible spirit.

$19.99

ORDER NOW

Gloria Hendry's Latest Masterpiece, The newest book is a compelling exploration of ambition, resilience, and self-discovery. Gloria Hendry, a young woman striving for success, embarks on a journey where love, excellence, free will, and truth serve as guiding forces. As she navigates life's challenges, she comes to an important realization: her ability to handle adversity directly impacts the heights she can reach. Hendry's storytelling is both heartfelt and insightful, offering a deeply human perspective on the pursuit of greatness. The novel skillfully weaves emotional depth with philosophical reflections, leaving readers with a renewed appreciation for the interplay between struggle and triumph. Her experiences resonate with anyone who has faced obstacles in their path to achievement.

One of the book's greatest strengths is its ability to inspire. Readers are not just taken on the protagonist's journey—they are encouraged to reflect on their own aspirations and the hurdles they must overcome. The novel is beautifully written, with engaging prose that keeps the pages turning. An inspiring read, rich with wisdom and emotional resonance. It is a must-read for anyone seeking motivation and a deeper understanding of how perseverance shapes success.

Paperback & KINDLE
100 pages   English   September 2022   8.5 x 0.26 x 11 inches

AVAILABLE ON AMAZON.COM

TRADITIONAL NG GA KUEN
KUNG FU

MASTER ANGEL VELAZQUEZ

"Whispers of the Furious Tiger"
ONE ON ONE TRAINING OR GROUP
OPEN SEMINARS
GET YOUR COPY TODAY

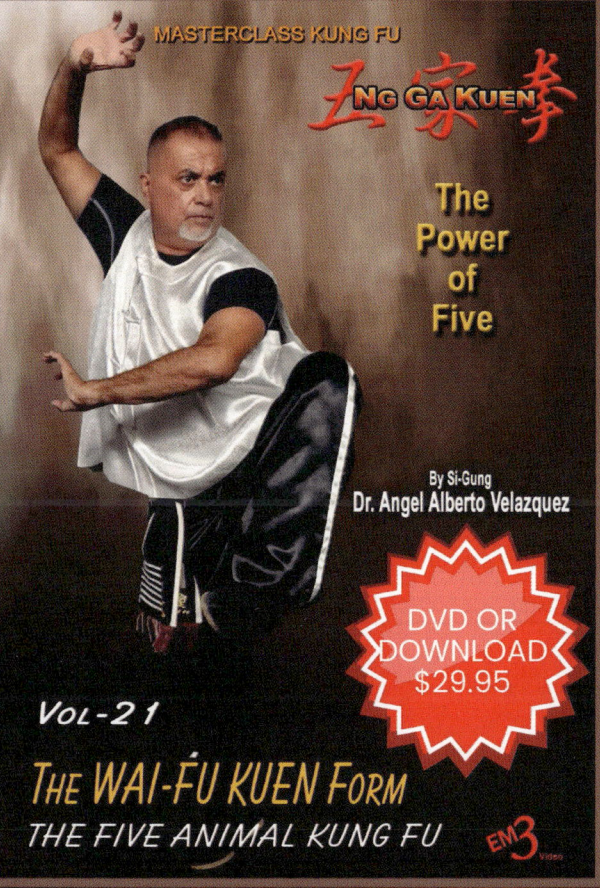
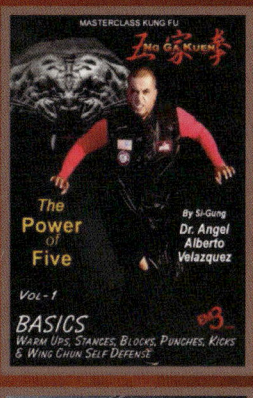
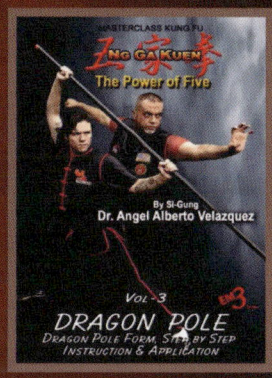
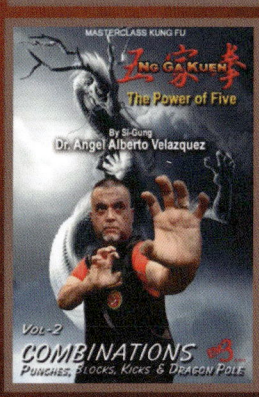
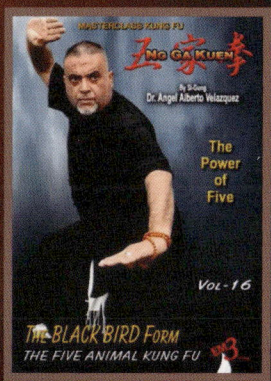

DVD OR DOWNLOAD $29.95

WITH EXPERT INSTRUCTION AND COMPREHENSIVE TECHNIQUES, YOU'LL GAIN THE SKILLS AND CONFIDENCE TO EXCEL IN YOUR PRACTICE.

Whether you're training at home or in class, these DVDs are designed to elevate your ability and deepen your understanding of this powerful art.

ORDER TODAY OR BOOK YOUR SEMINARS

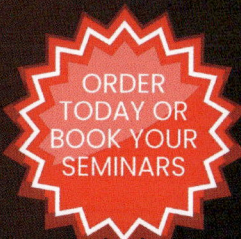

AngelsBlackTigerUSA@gmail.com for downloads

AngelsBlackTigerUSA@gmail.com to get your direct mail order today

CYNTHIA ROTHROCK

FRESH FROM
BLACK CREEK

By Sumiko Nakano

In a dusty makeshift town that smells like blood, gunpowder, and old regrets, a woman walks through the grit like she owns the place—because, frankly, she does. She's not twenty. She doesn't need to be. Her eyes don't flinch, her spine doesn't bend, and when a hulking outlaw steps up to test her, he ends up kissing the dirt after she slams him with a scorpion kick sharp enough to slice through time. Cynthia Rothrock, sixty-seven years young and still handing out beatings like it's the 1980s. And the crew? They break into applause. Because what they just witnessed isn't just another fight scene—it's history flexing its muscles.

Again.

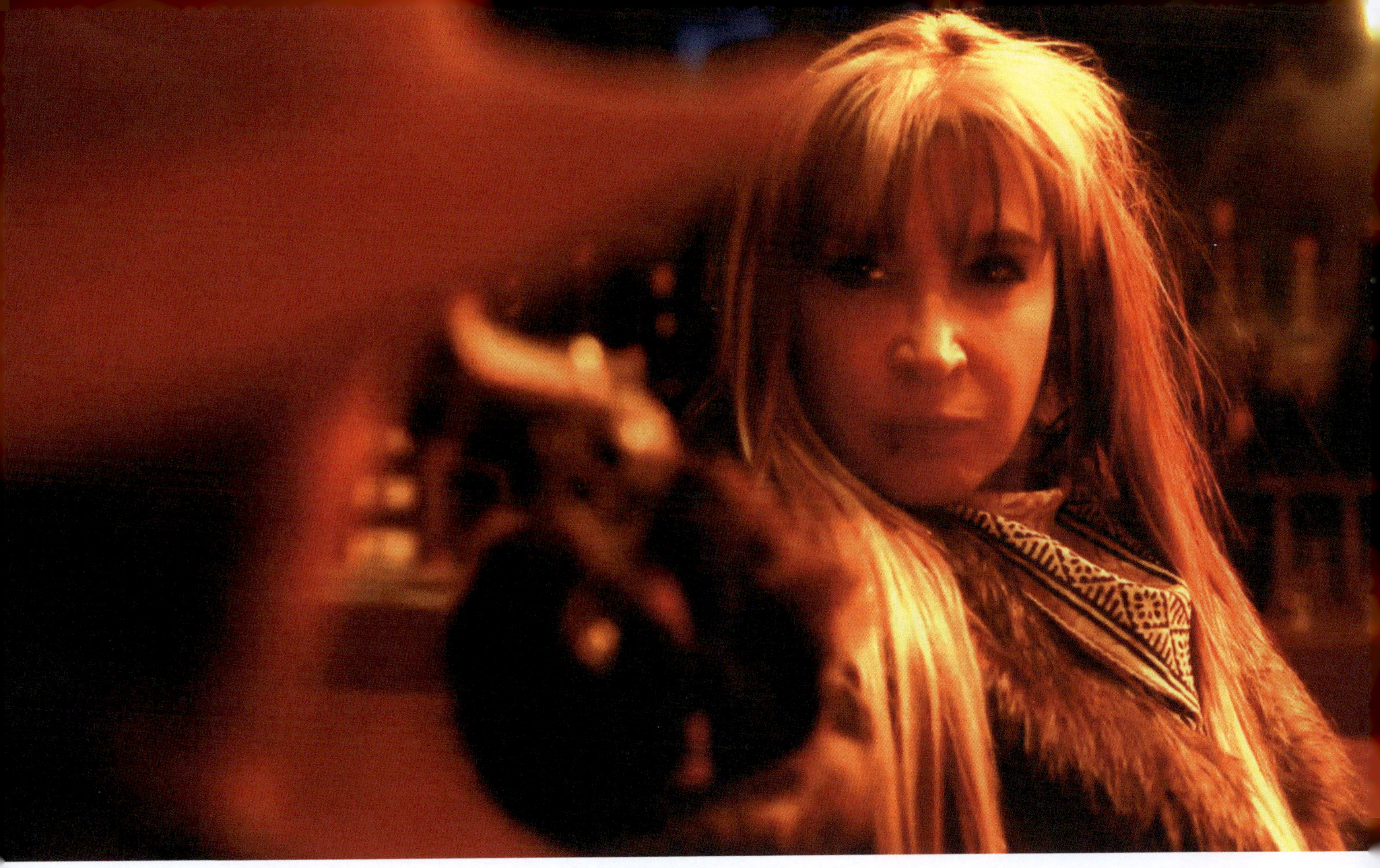

This is Black Creek, a western with dust in its teeth and fire in its chest. And Rothrock isn't just acting in it—she's rewriting the whole narrative. Not just of the film, but of her own legacy. Because this isn't a comeback story. She never left.

She was just waiting for a role worthy of everything she's learned, every bone she's broken, every lie she's shattered about what women can and can't do in this game.

Before she became the cowboy riding into justice with both fists cocked and a six-shooter on her hip, Cynthia Rothrock had already done what most people only dream of: beat the system at its own game.

Born in small-town Pennsylvania in 1957, she wasn't the prodigy the movies love to romanticize. She was the girl who chose the grind.

She walked into her first martial arts class at 13 and never looked back. Tang Soo Do, Taekwondo, Eagle Claw, Northern Shaolin—she didn't just dabble, she dominated. And in the cutthroat world of late-70s martial arts tournaments—where women were expected to smile, not fight—Rothrock showed up, showed out, and shut it all down.

Five-time undefeated world champion in forms and weapons from 1981 to 1985. That wasn't just unheard of—it was unthinkable.
But here's what made her dangerous: it wasn't just about winning. It was about making a statement.

That women don't need permission to take up space. That skill has no gender. And that if you put a sword in her hand or lined her up across from your best fighter, she was walking out the winner, clean and silent.

She didn't just earn respect. She demanded it, one broken expectation at a time.

The trophies weren't enough. The spotlight wasn't the goal. The fight was always the thing.

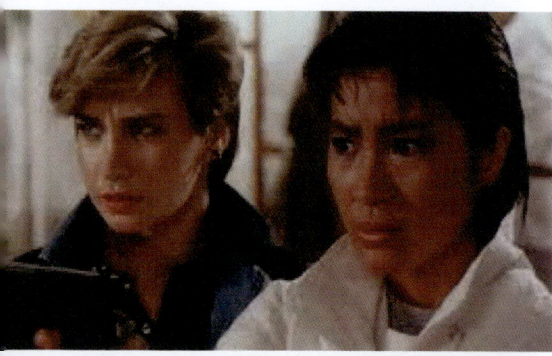

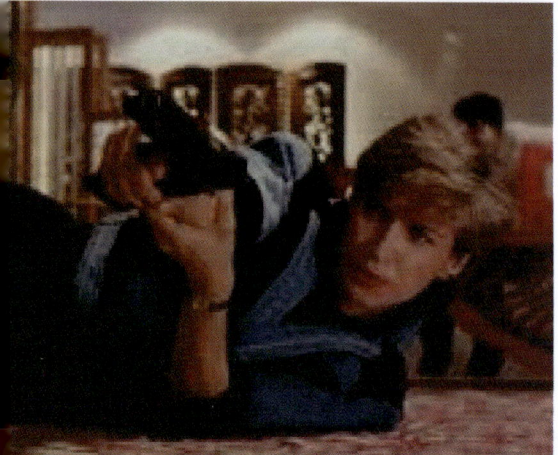

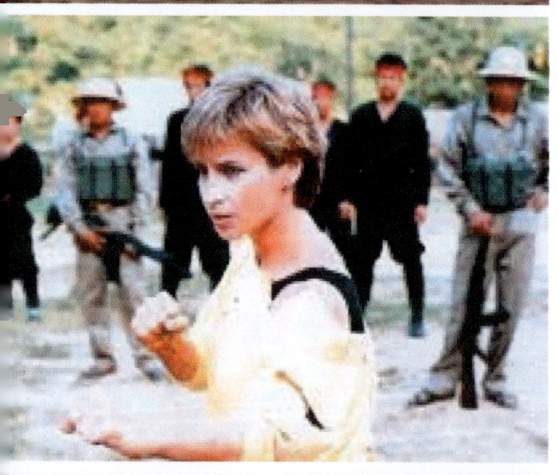

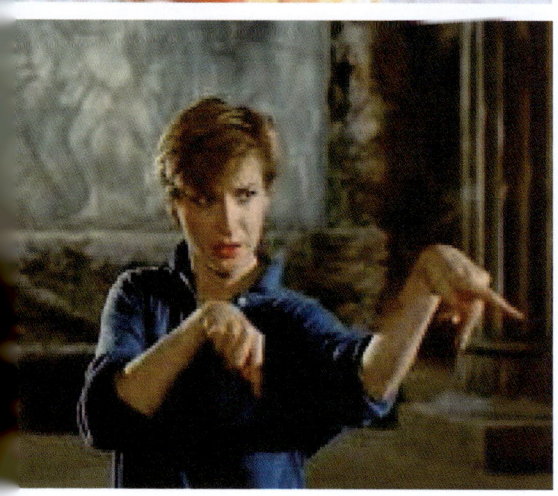

That mindset led her straight to the unlikeliest battlefield of all—Hong Kong. 1985.

Back when being a blonde American woman in a Hong Kong action film was about as common as unicorns with black belts.

They cast her opposite Michelle Yeoh in Yes, Madam!, thinking it would be novel. What they didn't count on was Rothrock stealing every frame with kicks that looked like poetry and hit like conviction. Glass flew. Gangsters fell. Audiences cheered. And Cynthia Rothrock became the first non-Asian woman to headline in Hong Kong action cinema.

She didn't just fit in—she raised the bar.

There, under the brutal expectations of Golden Harvest Studios, Rothrock refined her screen fighting to something vicious and almost elegant.

No wires. No ego. Just skill, sweat, and the willingness to throw herself—literally—into walls, tables, and down staircases if it meant getting the shot.

With films like Righting Wrongs, Magic Crystal, and Shanghai Express, she didn't just earn her place in the boys' club—she ran it.

She made it impossible to ignore what women could do in action films. She didn't "pave the way." She ripped the road open with her bare hands and left a blueprint stained with grit and brilliance.

Hollywood noticed. And—unsurprisingly—had no idea what to do with her.

By the time she brought her talents back to the States, major studios were still hesitating to hand female fighters the lead.

Rothrock didn't wait for a nod. She carved out her place in the independent action world—the core of martial arts cinema—where skill mattered more than budget and attitude outweighed polish.

If mainstream Hollywood was busy playing it safe, Cynthia was busy making impact. China O'Brien, Lady Dragon, Martial Law, Tiger Claws—her VHS covers weren't just box art. They were promises.

Fast hands. Fierce presence. No apologies.

She made fight scenes feel honest.

No slow-mo distractions, no choreography masking weakness. Just her and anyone bold enough to step in frame.

She didn't chase celebrity. She built trust. Audiences knew she could actually fight. And in a genre where authenticity is everything, she became iconic.

Not because she was handed it, but because she kept showing up and holding the line. She never stopped moving forward. And she still isn't.

When martial arts films gave way to superheroes and spectacle, the industry shifted—most fighters either adapted or disappeared. Cynthia Rothrock? She evolved. Quietly. Strategically. On her terms.

The films kept coming. One a year, steady. No need to announce it or shout into the void.

She was still working, still performing, still leading—just not chasing attention. Instead, she doubled down on something deeper: teaching.

She became what few action stars ever become—an actual master. Not just of movement, but of message.

Her seminars weren't for show. They were for the next generation of fighters.

The kind who might never get a studio break but would leave with something real. Precision. Strength. Self-respect. And wherever she went, people still called her Sensei. Not because of what she once did. Because of what she still does.

She wasn't chasing fame anymore. She was investing in legacy. The kind you don't build on a screen—you build on the mat.
In sweat.
In scars.

In a student's eyes when they realize they don't have to shrink to survive.

She didn't disappear. She just chose her lane. And when Black Creek happened, it wasn't a return. It was the next move in a long game she's been playing better than anyone.

Black Creek wasn't just another "project." It was war paint. A Western, yes, but one dragged through the dirt, loaded with pain, fury, and justice.

She didn't just star in it. She helped build it. Produced it. Funded it. Controlled it. Because Rothrock's not interested in being cast anymore.

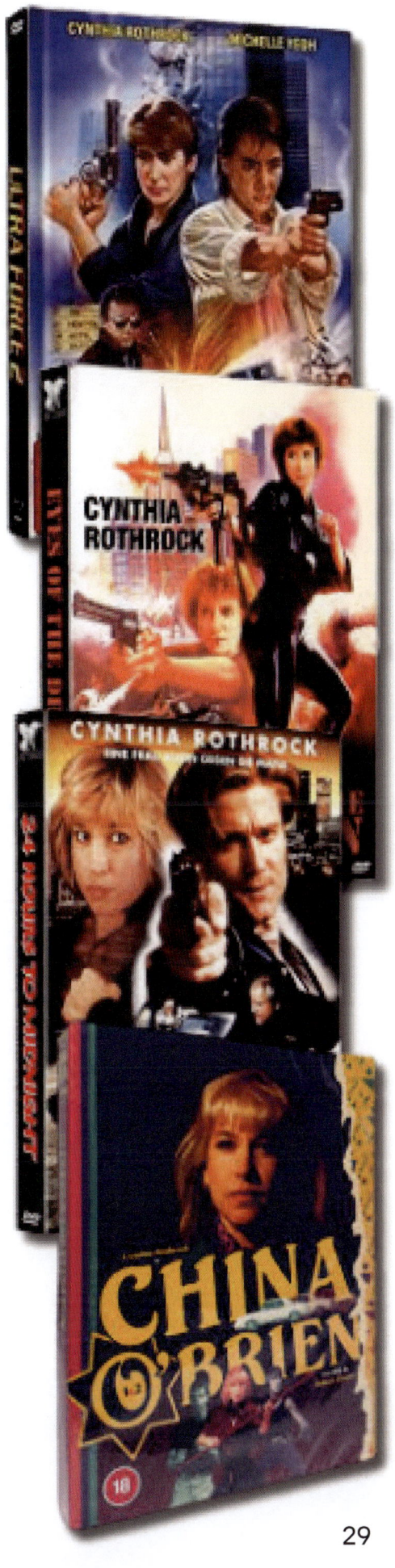

May 2025 / Vol. 2 - No. 5

She's interested in creating. And this time, she made a film where her character Ember doesn't need permission to be powerful, broken, dangerous, or human. She just is.

Ember is vengeance in a dusty coat. She's a woman who's lost too much to be gentle and seen too much to be naïve. And Rothrock gives her that lived-in weight—the kind of pain that doesn't beg for sympathy, just space to breathe and the freedom to retaliate.

Ember picks up a badge not out of hope, but out of duty. She doesn't cry in alleyways or lean on someone to fix her. She straps on the tools of justice and finishes what needs finishing.

That's not fiction. That's Cynthia.

When the fighting starts? It's still precise. Still brutal. No wasted motion. No ego. Just that same terrifying clarity that made her a world champion all those years ago.

A barstool becomes a launchpad. A scorpion kick becomes punctuation. And the point is made.

She hasn't lost anything. She's just gotten sharper.

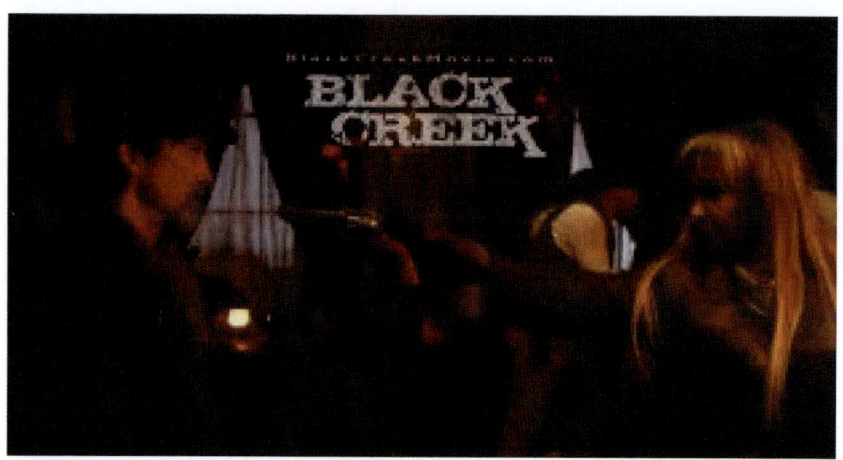

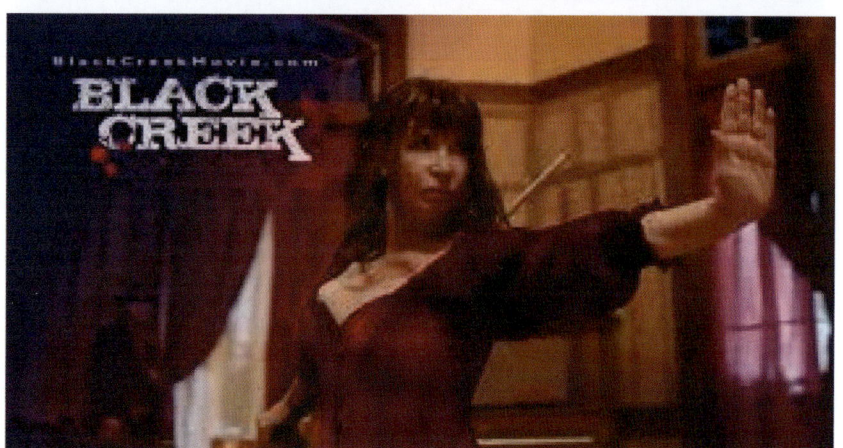

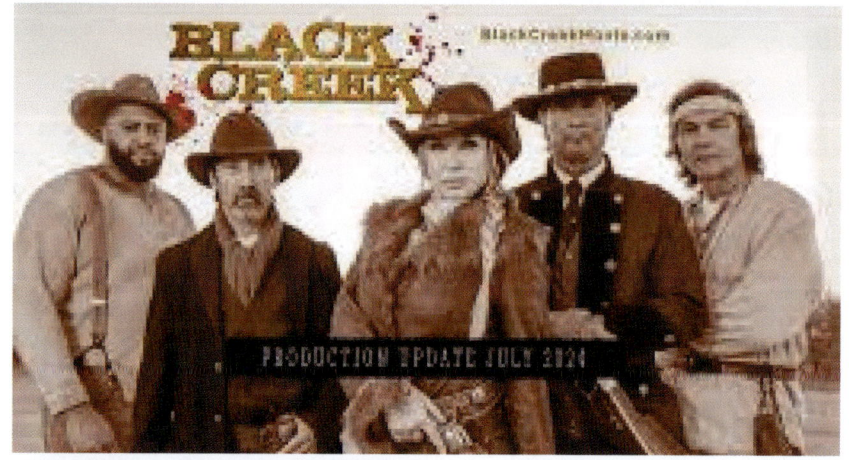

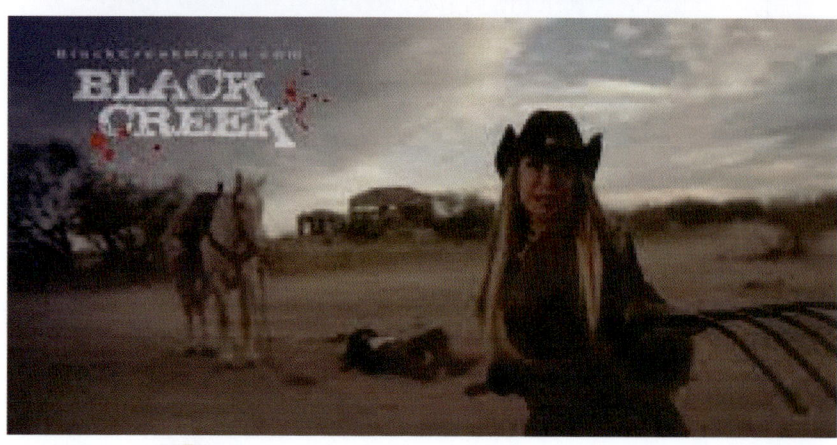

Black Creek isn't her return. It's her evolution. Rothrock doesn't play Ember as someone clinging to past glories. She plays her like someone who's still in the fight —and always has been.

There's no performance here. Just the truth. Experience in her bones. Steel in her stare. And that rare ability to carry weight without saying a word. She's not proving anything. She doesn't have to. The question isn't whether she still belongs—it's who will try and stand in her way.

Now, let's talk about the acting, because Black Creek doesn't just let her hit. It lets her feel. Ember's grief isn't scripted. It's lived in.

It's in the silence. The hesitation before a door. The way her fingers close around her brother's badge like a promise.

Rothrock doesn't play tough. She plays honest. For those of us who've been watching for decades, it's something deeper than ever before. It's human. Maybe it's her most dangerous work yet. Because it reminds you—she's not just a fighter. She's a storyteller.

You can feel every year she's earned. And every lesson she's carried. Ember doesn't posture.

She acts. Every step is calculated. Every strike has meaning. It's not about spectacle. It's about impact.

Rothrock doesn't chase legacy. She is legacy.

Watching Black Creek feels like watching her entire career ride through that canyon one more time.

The teenager in Pennsylvania. The fearless lead in Hong Kong. The undisputed queen of the home video martial arts boom. The teacher. The builder. The woman behind her own camera. And now— this.

Ember. Another chapter written by her own hand. She didn't wait for the industry to notice. She reminded it who taught it how to swing.

So no—this isn't a "comeback." Cynthia Rothrock didn't come back. She waited. Then she chose her moment. And she made it count.

She never left.

When Black Creek fades out and Ember rides into that molten sky, it might look like an ending. But you'd be wrong. Because Rothrock's not done. She's already training. Already thinking. Already planning the next one. Another film. Another genre. Another chance to prove—quietly, relentlessly—that the fire never went out.

Because you can't erase what built itself from nothing. And you definitely can't silence someone who's never needed to shout.

Cynthia Rothrock doesn't need to be remembered. She's still writing the story, and it's still landing with impact.

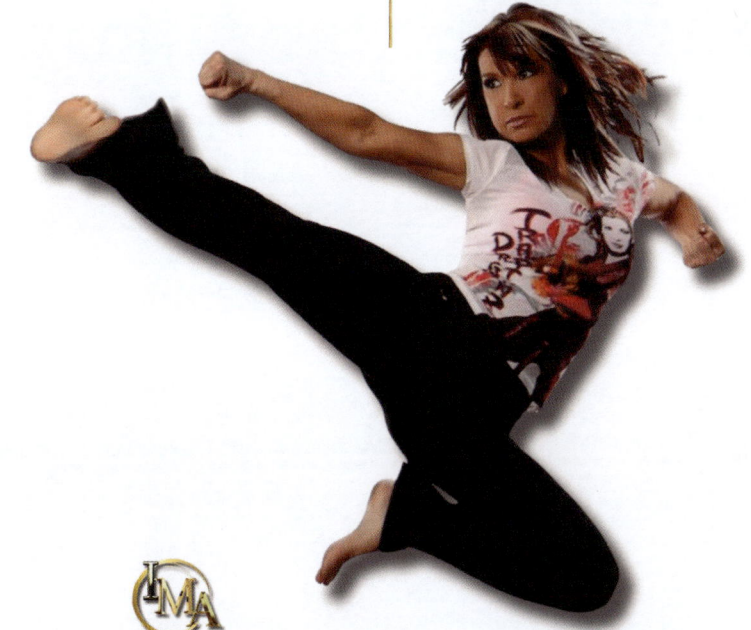

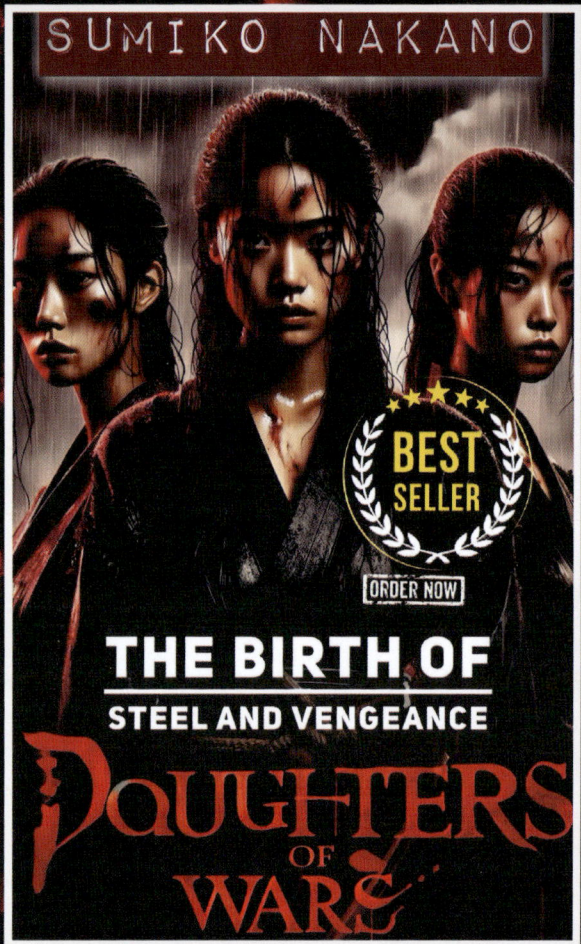

Step into the world of "Daughters of Wars," a historical fiction series that explores the lives of the Hayashi sisters during Japan's tumultuous shift from the Tokugawa shogunate to the Meiji Restoration.

The story follows the Hayashi sisters as they confront the challenges brought on by the Emperor's advancing forces, their own familial responsibilities, and the restrictive societal roles expected of women. Each sister brings unique strengths to their family's mission

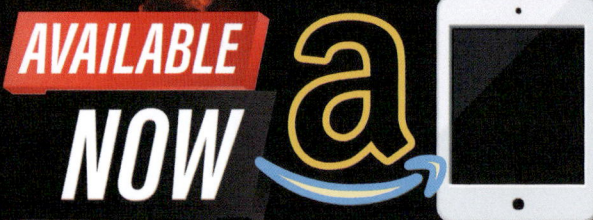

$6.99
AVAILABLE ON AMAZON.COM

HOJOJUTSU
VOL 1-2 BOOK & DVD

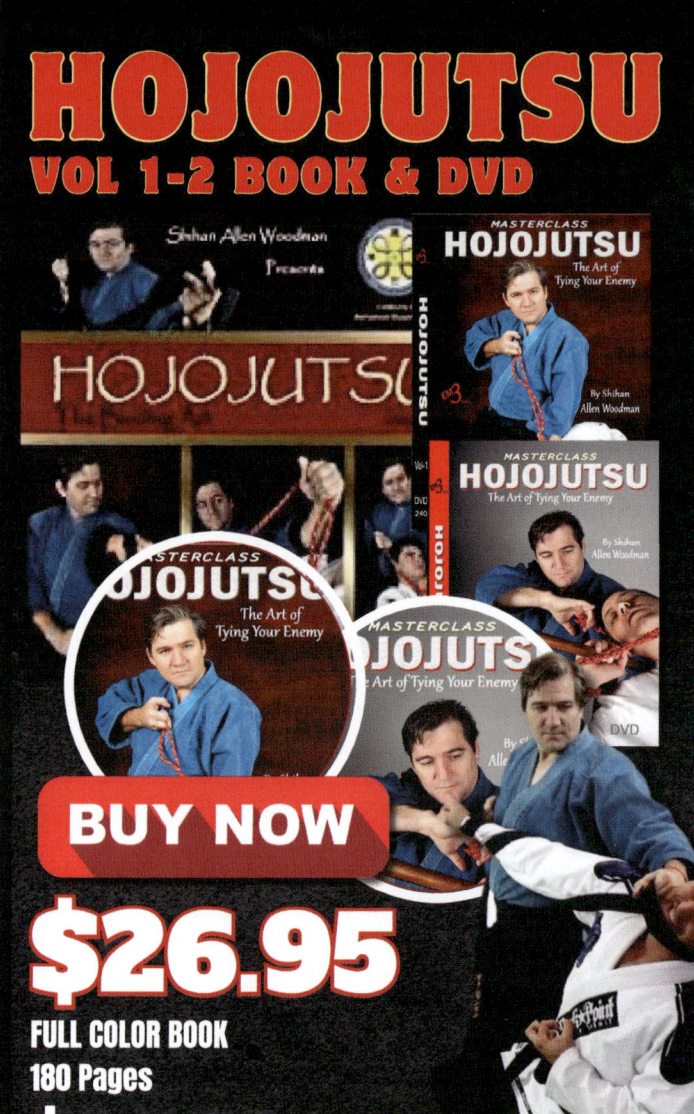

BUY NOW

$26.95
FULL COLOR BOOK
180 Pages

$14.95 Each DVD
The Art of Tying Your Enemy
DVD 1 & 2   47 min.

Hojojutsu is a traditional Japanese martial art of restraining that encompasses different school techniques. It is a unique product of Japanese history and culture and is rarely practiced outside Japan. It is part of the curriculum under the aegis of bugei and in jujutsu. There are very few videos or books available on this art. Shihan Allen Woodman teaches you hands-on each technique in a step-by-step format.

AVAILABLE ON AMAZON.COM

Bests Selling Books by Bohdi Sanders

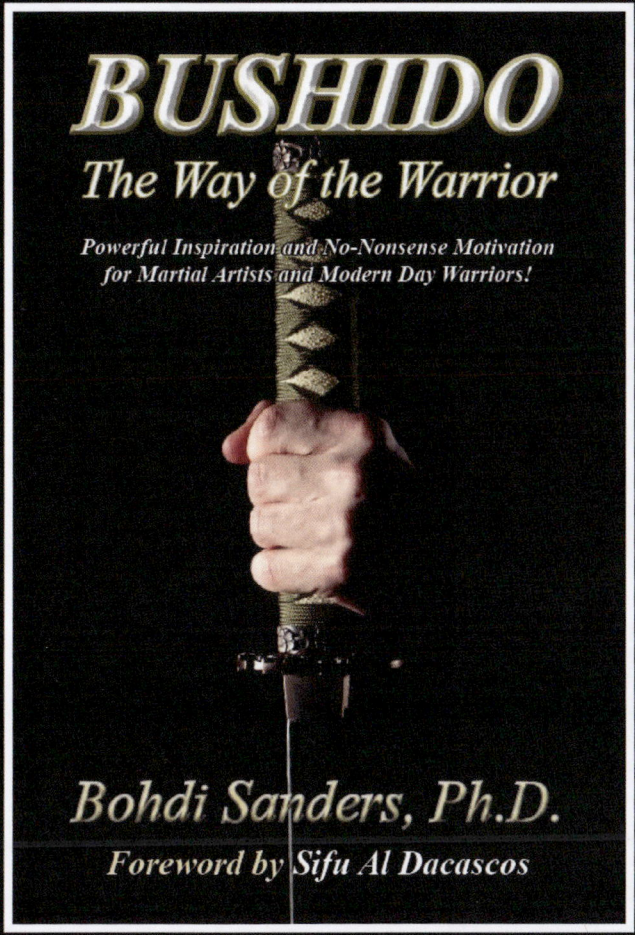
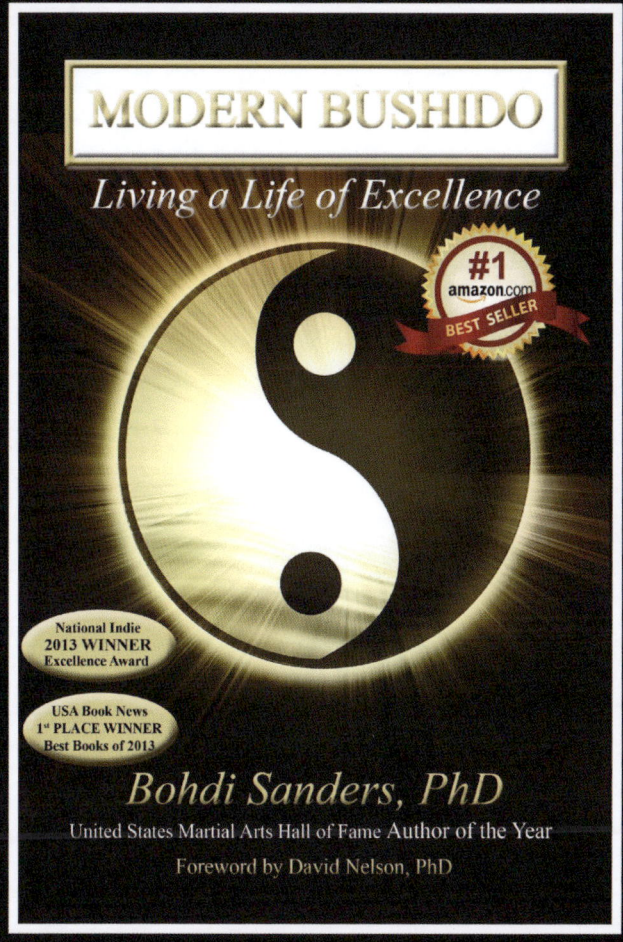

Check Out The PACKAGE DISCOUNTS and SAVE BIG!
Discount Packages Now Available on TheWisdomWarrior.com!

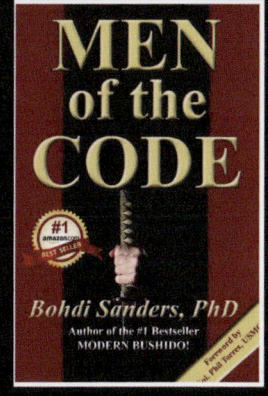
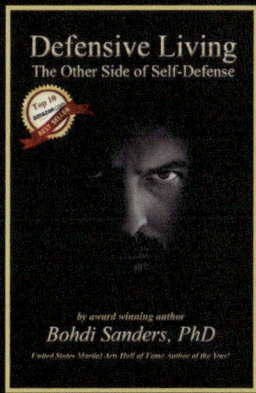
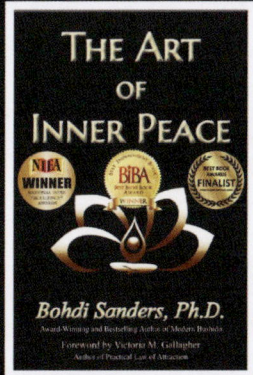
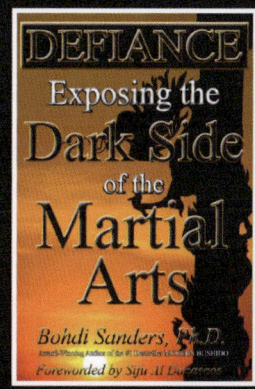
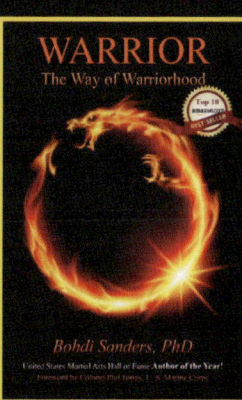

All of Shihan Sanders' Books are Available on:
TheWisdomWarrior.com and on Amazon.com!
GET YOUR COPIES TODAY!!

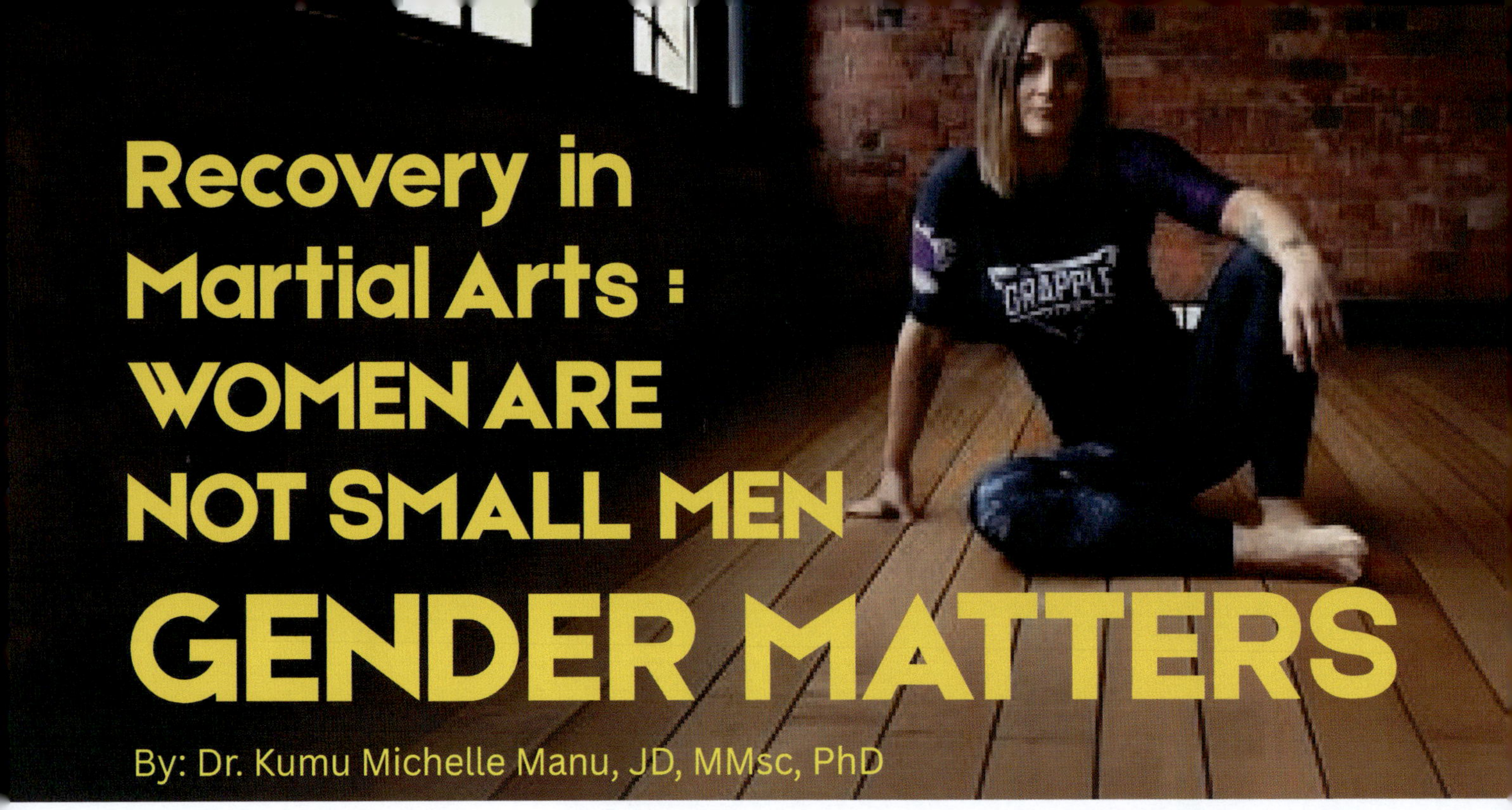

Recovery in Martial Arts: WOMEN ARE NOT SMALL MEN GENDER MATTERS

By: Dr. Kumu Michelle Manu, JD, MMsc, PhD

Women's health benefits in martial arts recovery include improved nutrition, quicker recovery periods, and enhanced immune system support. Martial arts also offer opportunities for personal growth, confidence building, and self-defense skills, promoting mental and emotional well-being.

In martial arts culture, recovery is often seen as secondary or optional - a silent and unglorified process expected to happen in the background. The stoic warrior limps off the mat, saying nothing. We are praised for "pushing through" the pain, not for listening to it.

This mindset is not only outdated; it's dangerous. I've seen too many high-level practitioners burn out, lose function, suffer long-term health consequences, or quit altogether because they never learned how to recover strategically, consistently, and appropriately for their body and level of training.

True recovery is a discipline of its own, one that requires self-awareness, humility, and often a complete emotional and identity shift.

"Martial arts should be about lifelong practice, not burnout and breakdown."

Women Are Not Small Men

The recovery process for women is fundamentally different than for men. Our hormonal rhythms, connective tissue composition, and injury patterns demand unique strategies. Yet, most recovery protocols are designed for men and applied to women without adaptation. For example:

- Hormones affect recovery windows. Estrogen supports joint laxity and tissue repair, but its fluctuations can make women more prone to soft tissue injuries depending on their cycle.

- Women often experience different injury patterns, such as ACL tears, due to structural and neuromuscular differences.

- Postpartum recovery is rarely addressed in martial arts circles, even though many female martial artists continue training during or soon after pregnancy.

These physiological differences should not be sidelined; they should be studied, embraced, and addressed with intention.

Age Matters: The Warrior Evolves

- Our bodies are not static. A 25-year-old male fighter and a 50-year-old woman master have profoundly different recovery needs. Yet, most training models fail to account for this.

- Recovery shifts with age: Sleep becomes more essential and more elusive.

- Tendon elasticity decreases, requiring more time to warm up and cool down.

- Inflammation takes longer to resolve, and overtraining even more destructive.

- Mental focus may sharpen, but physical resiliency may decrease – meaning smarter, not harder training is required.

- Cold recovery for young men. Heat recovery for women of all ages.

For seasoned martial artists entering their elder years, recovery isn't about "bouncing back." It's about strategically staying in the game at our highest level.

"What's the point of mastering combat if you can't move at 50, 60, or 70?"

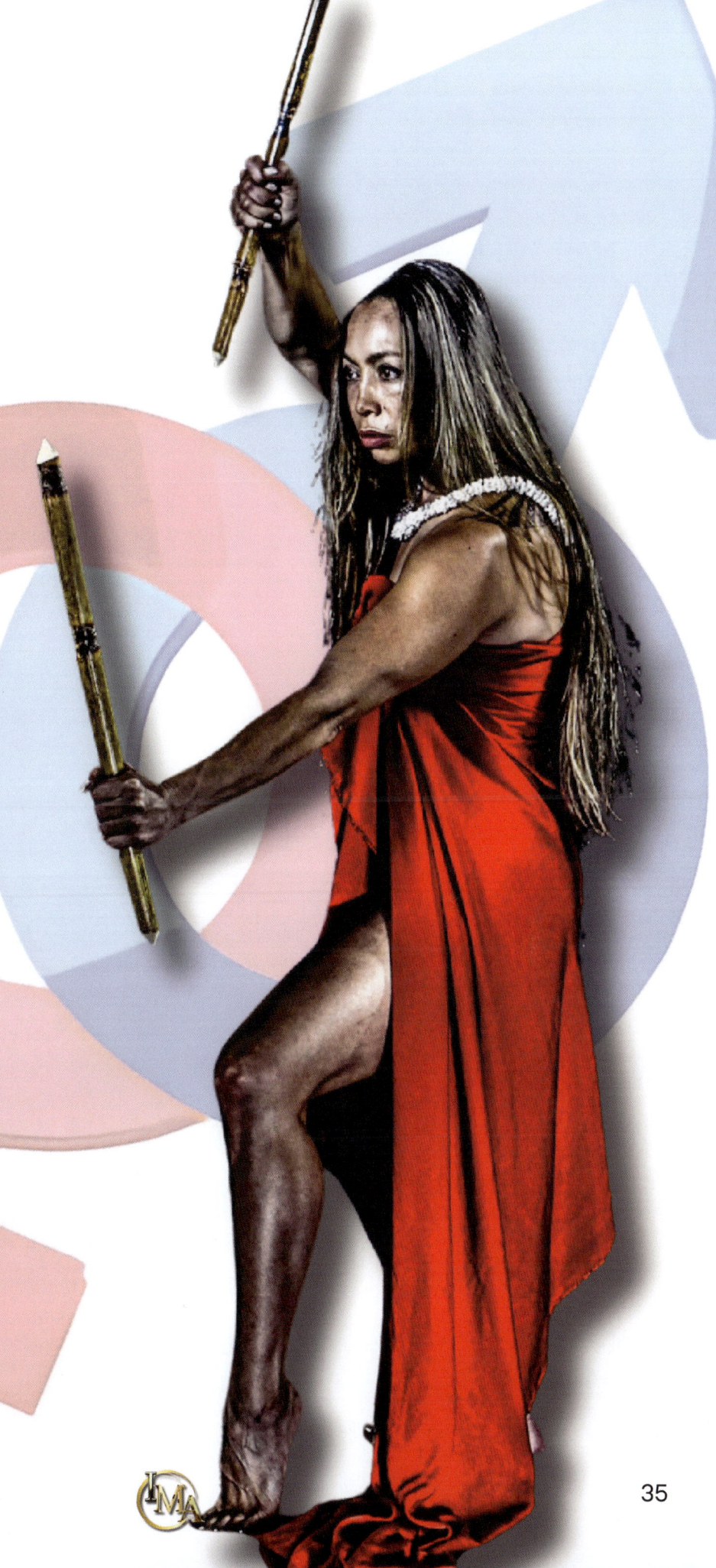

The Warrior Woman Over 40: Recovery as Sacred

As I recover from yet another major surgery, one that forced me to pause all physical practice and teaching -

I have come face-to-face with the vulnerability many warriors try to avoid.

I've had to redefine strength.
I've had to allow others to see me still, limited, and in transition.
That alone was a lesson in warrior humility.

"Rest by choice, or your body will choose for you."

Rest isn't just about stillness. It is about gently and powerfully returning to your why.
Why are you a martial artist?
Why do you fight?
Why do you dedicate your life to this path?

Ancient Hawaiian Warriors: Recovery as Ritual

Kanaka Maoli/Ancient Hawaiian warriors (nā koa) understood what many modern warriors have forgotten:

Rest and recovery were not separate from battle - they were part of the training cycle.

Elite Lua warriors were trained in bone setting - not just to dislocate their enemies' joints in combat, but to reset their fellow warriors' injuries on the battlefield. They were also trained in plant medicine, warrior massage, and ocean therapy to heal wounds, relieve pain, and strengthen the body.

Unlike modern warriors who often see rest as weakness, Hawaiians viewed it as a necessary rhythm that kept the warrior body, mind, and spirit in balance. A warrior who does not rest cannot fight.

"Ho'omaha, a laila e ho'i hou i ke kaua."

Rest, then return to battle.

They didn't just recover physically; they also knew that mental and emotional restoration and balance was critical.

They released the emotional burdens from battle, restored their mana (spiritual power) if it had been weakened, and ensured their minds and hearts were clear before returning to combat.
of body text

a warrior carrying mental or emotional instability into battle was considered a liability to their ali'i (chief) and fellow warriors. Recovery was a necessity for survival. Healing is not just physical; it requires spiritual balance.

"E ola ka 'uhane, ola ke kino."
 When the spirit is well, the body is well.

Michelle Manu

ABOUT THE AUTHOR

Michelle Manu is a groundbreaking figure—**an elite Hawaiian Lua warrior, lifelong athlete, legal executive, metaphysician, and public figure dedicated to warrior training, cultural preservation, and women's empowerment**.

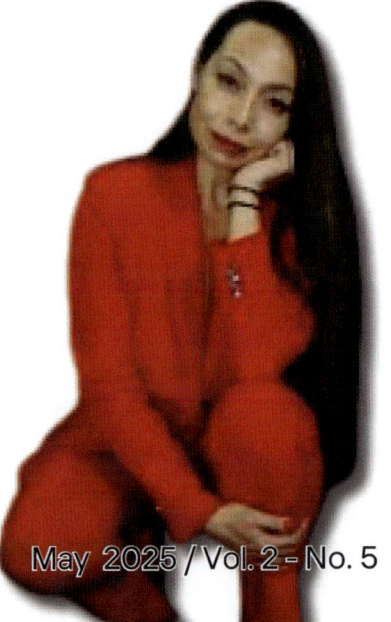

BIG SALE
GET UP TO 30% OFF

APPLY DIRECLY FOR A FULL YEAR SUBSCRIPTION

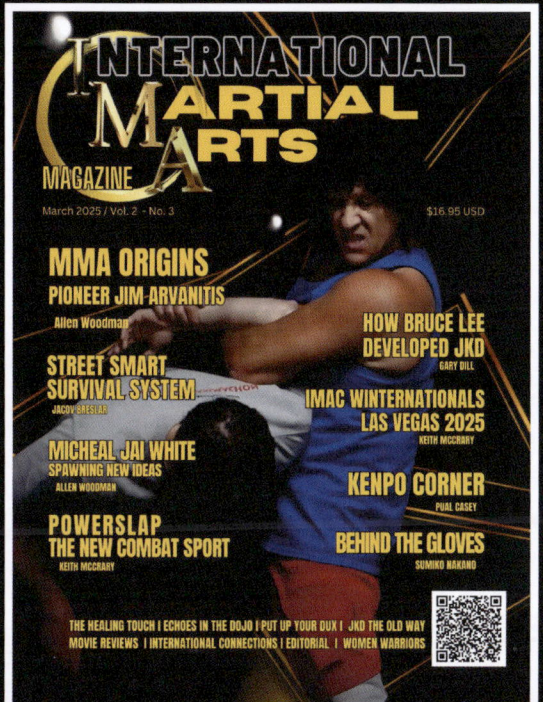
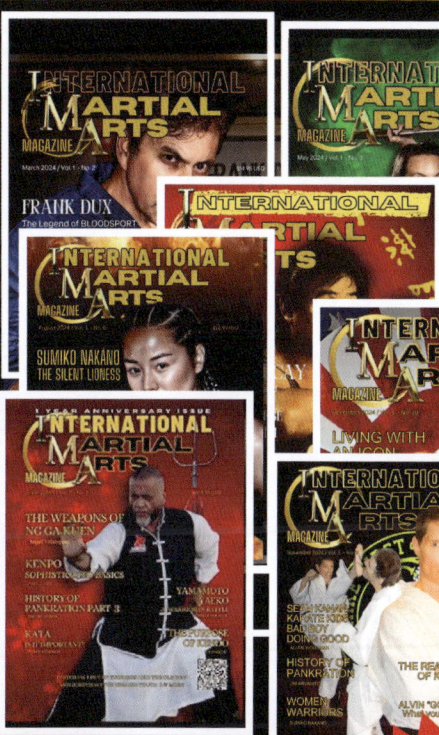

MONTHLY INDUSTRY MAGAZINE

International Martial Arts Magazine is a NEW Monthly magazine focused on all the various aspects of martial arts. With fascinating and riveting articles and featured stories along with columnists like the martial arts ICON Frank Dux of "Bloodsport" fame, Author Bohdi Sanders, Legendary instructor Gary Dill, and many more. Join us each month as we bring you all the excitement and information on the martial arts world around you. From traditional martial arts to new progressive theories and practices, this magazine allows you an inside look at the arts and the people that make them great. Join us for each issue. Contact us directly to apply for a yearly subscription. All orders must be paid in full to receive the annual 30% discount.

artseastpublish@gmail.com

ONLY $14.95 Per Issue

JOSHITAI
Unsung Heroines of the Boshin War

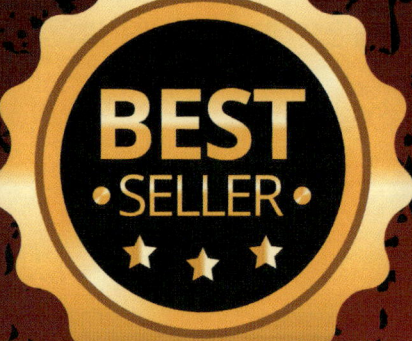

"The Jōshitai: Unsung Heroines of the Boshin War" by Sumiko Nakano is a concise yet powerful tribute to the brave women who played a pivotal role during one of Japan's most transformative periods.
This book offers a brief overview of the lives and contributions of 19 courageous women warriors, from seasoned samurai to devoted family members, who stood firm during the Boshin War.

Led by the fearless Nakano Takeko, these women defied societal norms to defend their homeland against over-whelming odds.

Each chapter provides a summarized account of their bravery and strategic acumen, highlighting their commitment to their domain and families. While the book may not delve deeply into each woman's life, it serves to make their names known and honor their contributions.

Paperback & KINDLE

July 13, 2024
105 pages
English
6 x 0.24 x 9 inches

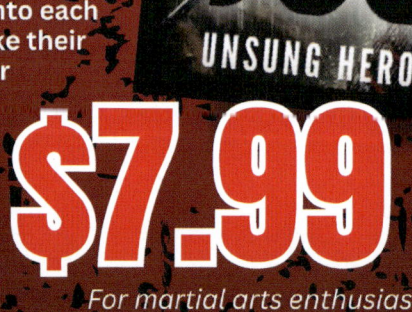

$7.99

ORDER NOW

For martial arts enthusiasts and history buffs alike, Joshintai is an unmissable treasure. Whether you're a seasoned practitioner or someone fascinated by the intricate tapestry of Japanese history, this book will leave you inspired and awestruck. Discover the extraordinary tales of these women whose legacies have been shrouded in shadows for far too long.

INTERNATIONAL MARTIAL ARTS MAGAZINE 2024

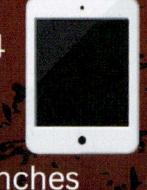

AVAILABLE ON AMAZON.COM

A Transformative Guide to *Personal Growth and Resilience*

- Demystify fear and pain: Explore their evolutionary roots and physiological effects.
- Master decision-making under duress.
- Build unshakable resilience: Cultivate mental toughness.
- Unlock the secrets of body bio-dynamics.
- Apply force ethically and responsibly.
- Recover, heal, and grow: Navigate the aftermath of conflict with strategies for physical recovery, emotional healing, and cultivating a positive mindset.

ORDER NOW

LIMITED TIME OFFER

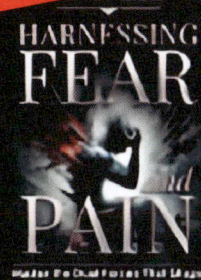
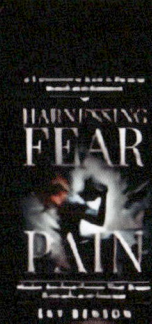

A Transformative Guide to *Personal Growth and Resilience*

HARNESSING FEAR and PAIN

Master the Dual Forces That Shape Strength and Courage

SKY BENSON

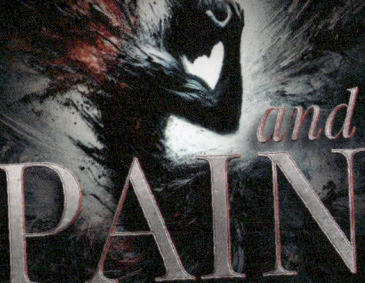

• SHOP NOW • SHOP NOW • SHOP NOW • SHOP NOW •

$19.95

Checkout more books on
www.vipublishing.com

AVAILABLE ON AMAZON.COM

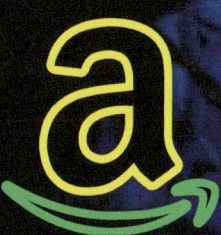

NATIONAL TOURNAMENT HITS HARD

By Keith McCrary

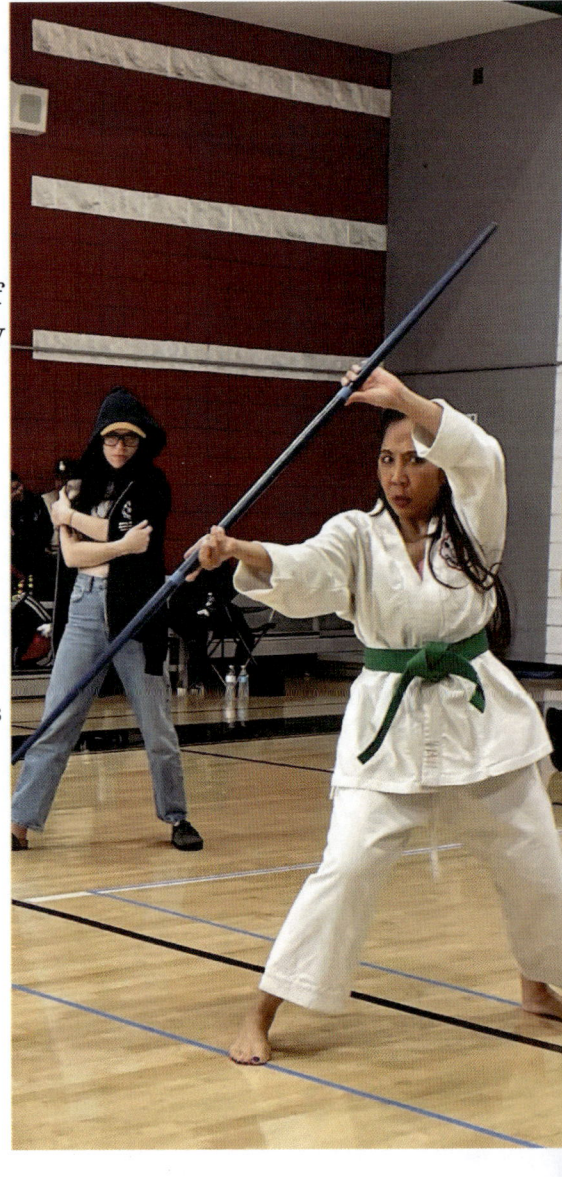

On April 6, 2023, Los Angeles, California, played host to a thrilling National Tournament that exceeded all expectations.

Initially, the promoters anticipated a light turnout, but to their surprise and delight, the event attracted an unexpectedly large crowd.

The vibrant atmosphere was palpable as martial artists of all ranks and ages gathered to compete in various divisions.

With several rings running simultaneously throughout the day, participants showcased their skills in fighting forms, weapons, and self-defense categories.

The diversity of competitors was impressive, with numerous schools from Mexico and surrounding cities in the greater L A. area

Martial arts schools very every corner of the city showed up, creating a rich tapestry of talent and tradition.

Among the attendees were our own editor and a group of giantesses, who were not only there to cover the event but were also drawn into the excitement and decided to participate.

Their involvement added a fun twist to the day, highlighting the inclusive spirit of the tournament. One of the standout performances came from MC Harshaw, a talented student and protégé of our editor.

Harshaw dominated the competition, winning gold medals in his black belt divisions, our Editor Allen Woodman also won in the Black belt self-defense and black belt weapons.

His remarkable skill and determination were a testament to the dedication and hard work that martial arts demand.

Competitors and spectators alike found the event to be fast-paced and friendly, fostering an environment of camaraderie and sportsmanship.

Despite the overwhelming attendance, the tournament wrapped up by 4 PM, a remarkable feat considering the number of participants. The success of this national-level event left everyone smiling and satisfied, showcasing the passion for martial arts that unites practitioners across different backgrounds.

As the day came to a close, it was clear that this tournament would be remembered not just for its scale, but for the joy and excitement it brought to all involved.

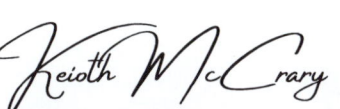

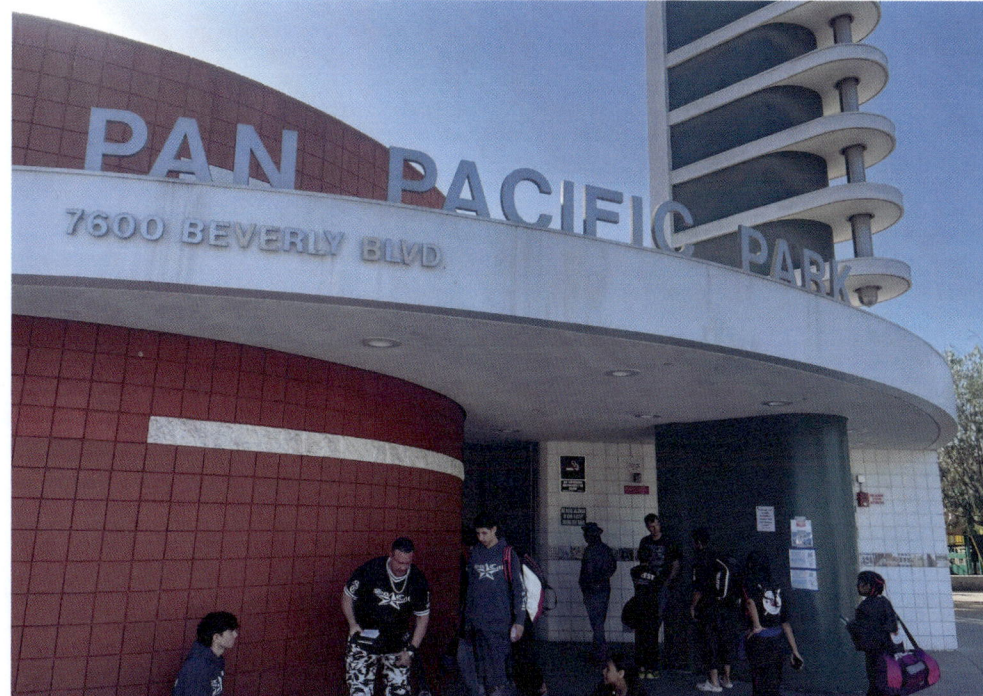

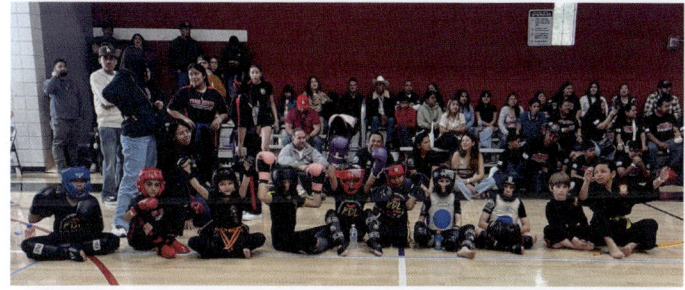

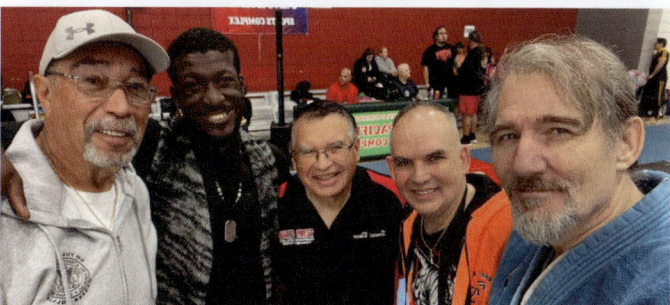

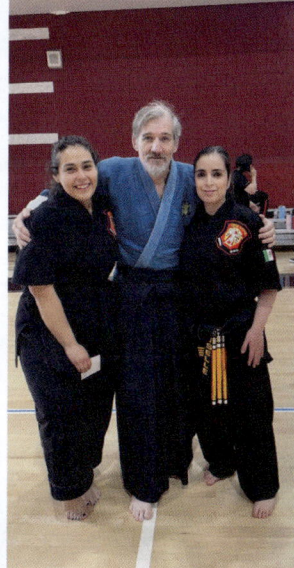

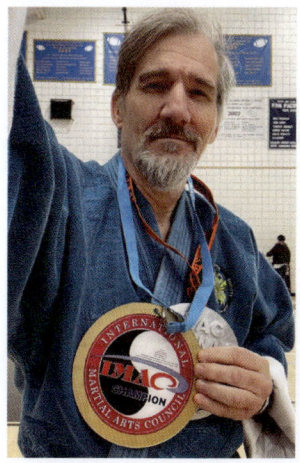
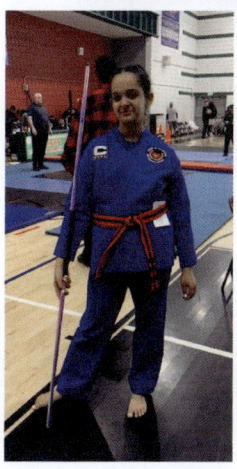
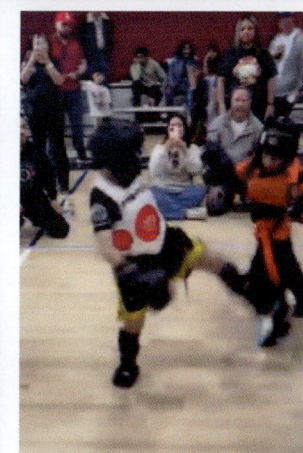
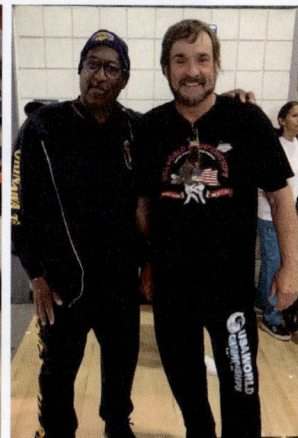
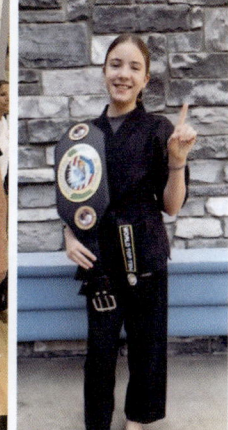

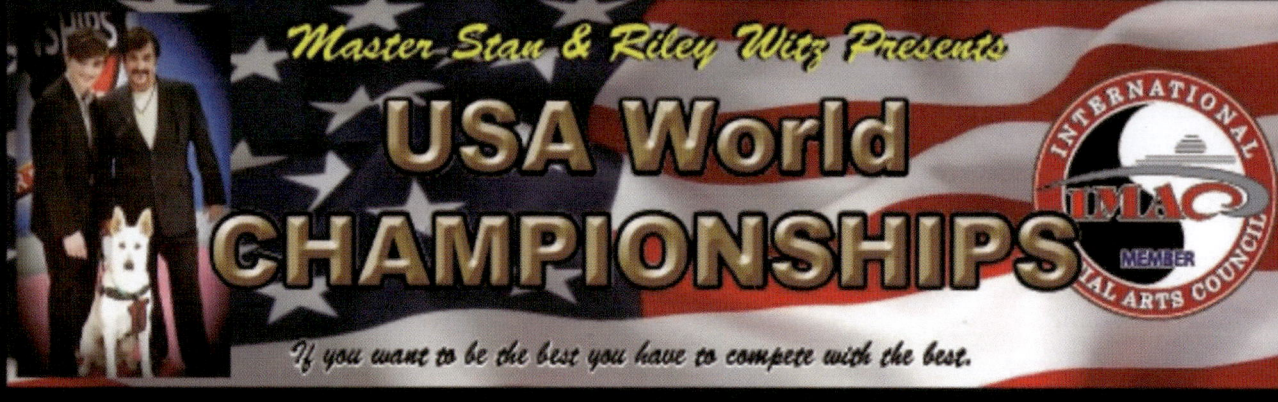

USA World CHAMPIONSHIPS

Master Stan & Riley Witz Presents

If you want to be the best you have to compete with the best.

JUNE 28, 29, 2025

The Orleans

To book your room at our special rates go to www.usaworldchampionships.com and click the book your room link.

DEMO TEAM WINNER WILL RECEIVE A CASH PRIZE

FRIST TIMER FORMS ARE FOR 13 YEARS AND UNDER WHITE, YELLOW, ORANGE ONLY

VEGAS

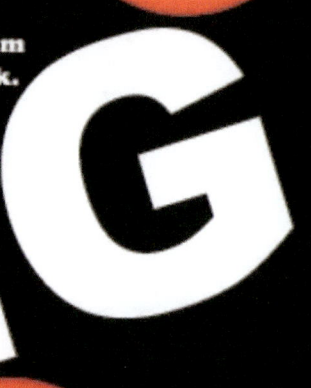

up to $1000 PROFESSIONAL POINT SPARRING

Each grand champion will receive a USA World Champion Ring

(702) 738-2507

usaworldchampionships.com

PANKRATION

MMA ORIGINS IN ANCIENT GREECE

Written By Jim Arvanitis

PART 6

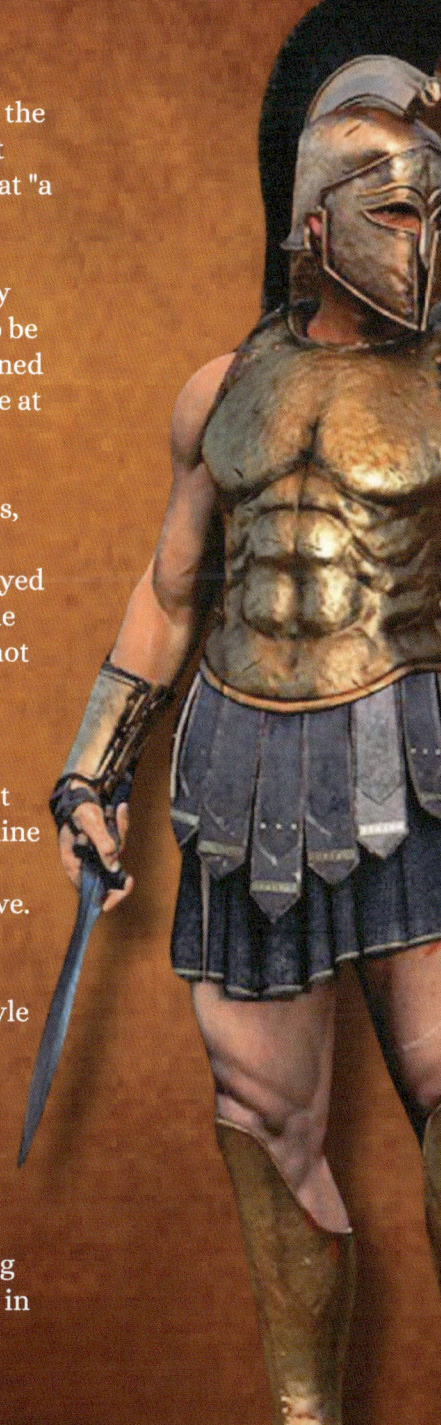

THE TRADITION

It's clear that the arms and armor of ancient Greece forged battle-ready warriors who possessed fearsome skills and indomitable spirits. For them there could be no retreat, no surrender.

The qualities on which they relied are perhaps best summed up in a message a Spartan mother gave her son as he went off to war: "E tan e epi tan." Its meaning – Return with your shield victorious … or carried home dead upon it.

Sparta was one of the foremost city-states in early Greek civilization. The Spartan army stood at its very core, and the primary obligation of citizens was to be good soldiers. Subject to military drilling from infancy, the Spartans were one of the most disciplined, well-trained and feared military forces in world history.

During Sparta's heyday in the 6th to 4th centuries B.C., it was generally accepted that "a single Spartan warrior equaled several from any other state." Their military education trained them to be survivors, and they remained undefeated until the Battle at Leuktra in 371 B.C.

Like the other Greek states, the Spartan army was infantry-based and employed the Phalanx formation. The Spartans themselves did not introduce any significant changes or tactical innovations in hoplite warfare, but their constant drilling and superb discipline made their phalanx much more cohesive and effective.

The Spartans used the phalanx in the classical style of a single line, uniformly deep in files of eight to twelve men.

The Spartans placed maximum importance on teamwork and maintaining the phalanx configuration in battle.

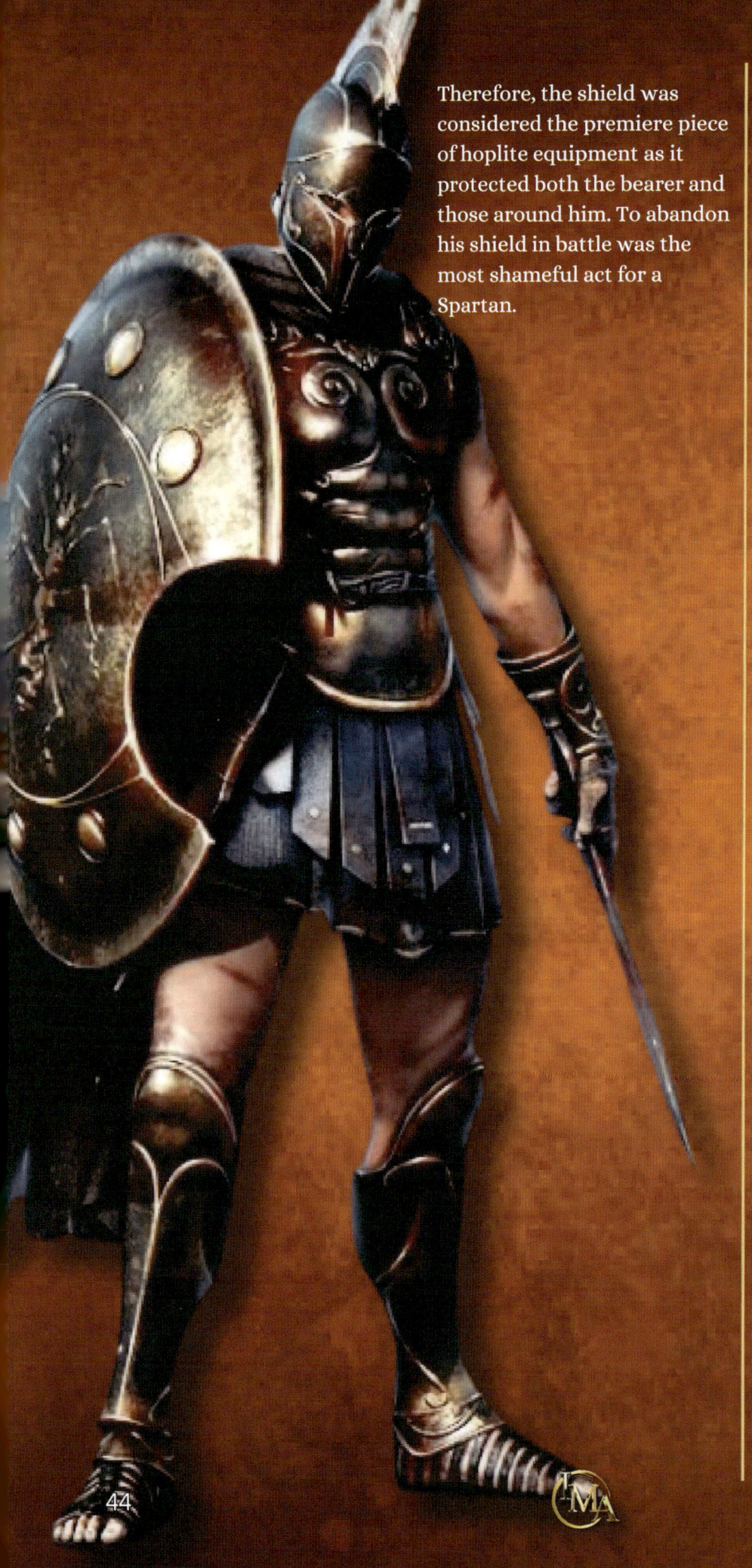

Therefore, the shield was considered the premiere piece of hoplite equipment as it protected both the bearer and those around him. To abandon his shield in battle was the most shameful act for a Spartan.

The Spartans used the same hoplite equipment as the other Greeks; the only distinctive features were the crimson tunic (chitōn) and cloak (himation), and the long hair, which the Spartans retained to a far later date than most Greeks. To the Spartans, the long hair retained its older Archaic meaning as the symbol of a free man.

Another widely known Spartan symbol, adopted in the mid-5th century B.C., was the letter lambda (Λ), standing for Lakonia or Lakedaemon, which was painted on their shields. Spartan hoplites were often portrayed bearing a transverse horsehair crest on their helmets, which was possibly used to identify officers.

Education was obligatory and uniform for all Spartan citizens. This enforced an important institutional restriction on the display of wealth unlike other Greek city-states, Athens in particular. Uniformity in training and learning was regulated through a system of Rites of Passage, which might be defined as rituals marking transitional phases in one's status in the context of social hierarchies, values, and beliefs. Sparta's most distinguished athletes were privileged to be included in the homoioi (the equals), which entitled them to fight in war alongside the king.

With their heavy emphasis on military strength and fitness, there are mythical claims that Spartan society practiced an institutional form of infanticide by throwing imperfect babies to their death off Mount Taygetus.

However, this is very likely a misconception attributed most often to the historical writings of Plutarch. He mentions that newborns were inspected by elders but this doesn't necessarily mean that those found to be unfit to serve later as soldiers were tossed to their demise.

The focus of Sparta's education was on producing ideal warriors through the agoge, a rigorous education and training regimen under the guardianship and control of the State. Boys were taken from their homes and families as early as age seven and were taught reading and writing for their basic needs.

The remainder of their instruction was dedicated to combat preparation. They were taught to obey orders and endure hardship without complaint, and grew up fearing disgrace more than death.

This did not confine the young men, however, to the harsh life of military existence. Some of its athletes took home the victory prizes from the earliest Olympiads.

Thucydides suggested that the Spartans were the first to introduce two innovations to the games and in training that became fundamental elements of Greek athletics – the complete nudity of the competitors and the covering of their bodies in oil.

The Spartans held religious and public festivals for competition between the different age groups. Their participation was compulsory and formed an official part of their training. Performance played a significant role in these rituals, and the kinetic and physical skills of the young Spartans were carefully accessed. One such festival, the Gymnopaidai, consisted of four dances which were designed as endurance tests.

Public floggings, sparse rations, and being forced to sleep outside in the cold were all part of a Spartan's training and conditioning. The philosopher Thucydides attests to the popular ritual of flagellations among the Lakedaemonians, claiming that those among them who could bear the greatest number of lashes acquired much glory for it.

It was used to test one's will and his ability to endure punishment, a quality of toughness called katereia.

Plato in his Laws underscored the importance of these ordeals as competitive games and the city of Sparta organized spectacles in which children and young men demonstrated their virtues and courage.

According to Pausanias, the early Spartans had a curious hazing contest in which groups of their young military trainees would be kept half-starved until they engaged in a public fight with each other over hunks of cheese on an altar.

The winner would get the food but also be declared the bomonikes (possibly a victor worthy of officer status), who had a statue erected in his honor or a large inscription of his name placed in a prominent area.

Much later, the endurance contest was changed to see which boy could endure a public whipping longest without crying uncle. In post-Hellenic times, after Rome had conquered the Greek city-states, this became a sort of bizarre tourist attraction, and Romans would come each spring and pay money to watch the Spartan youths flogged.

In the 3rd century A.D., the commercialized Spartans erected a theater around the altar.

At the festival of the goddess Artemus Ortheia, the older boys were required to participate in a competition where they had to snatch as much cheese as they could from the steps of the altar to the goddess.

They would have to pass through many guards armed with whips who were instructed to use them as forcefully as possible. Some of the youths died as a result.

Another brutal test was the agon rite (from which we get the English word "agony"), whereby the Spartan youths gathered outside during the hottest part of the year and at the hottest time of the day. They were stripped naked, basted with olive oil, and forced to dance for several hours under the blistering heat of the sun.

The dance was considered of extreme importance to the Spartans since in battle, they moved to the sound of musical signals.

They needed to learn to dance well so they could respond to these signals when engaged with the enemy. Those scant few who survived the agon were deemed fit and ready for service in the Spartan army.

Spartan Pankration

The militant Spartans practiced their own distinct brand of pankration and, like pammachon, it truly was no-holds-barred fighting.

Unlike that of the Eleans and the rest of the Greeks, there were no rules and it permitted EVERYTHING, even biting and gouging.

In his epigram, Philostratos commented that the "Spartans made war training for sport and sport training for war." He attributed the loss of the Spartans to the Thebans at the battle of Leuktra to the fact that the Thebans practiced more diligently in the palaestra. Plutarch, Lucian, and Philostratos also saw the connection between combat sport and hand-to-hand fighting.

Spartan athletes originally competed in Olympic wrestling and pankration and won many titles in both sports. They later discontinued due to a couple of reasons — they felt that the rules of the Olympic version, albeit two in number, were restrictive, and the fact that it was unacceptable for a Spartan to be defeated in physical combat at the hands of other Greeks.

To lose in running or a similar contest was seemingly condoned, however, and those from Lakedaemonia competed freely in such events. For a Spartan, the best place to utilize his pankration skills was in battle against enemy soldiers.

Combat sport trainers were a rarity, but when they became necessary, they were usually more knowledgeable in military tactics than the sporting aspect.

The focus was placed on valor rather than skill. The Spartan athletes exercised naked and outdoors in all types of weather and were subjected to routine hazing and abuse.

The Spartans were extremely reclusive and unwilling to permit outsiders on their lands, so little is known of their local pankration champions. The scant amount of information we have comes from the writings of Aristotle, Plutarch, and Herodotus, none of whom were of Spartan blood.

They tell us that Spartan pankration was, on the surface, consistent with the rest of Greece. However, there were some notable differences.

Their events were more of a violent nature than of good sportsmanship, and they favored group contests as opposed to individual matches (as was necessary in the phalanx formation).

Teams would compete on a remote island and aggressively strike, bite, and gouge with the objective of driving their targeted victim(s) into the water.

Part 7 Continues Next month

Jim Arvanitis

MMA ORIGINS

March 2025 / Vol. 2 - No. 3

ANCIENT GREEK MARTIAL ARTS: Warfare and Combat Sports in the Classical World is a fully illustrated guide to the battlefield tactics of the hoplite soldier and the athletic competitions that evolved from them. The author examines the heavy events of wrestling, boxing, and the all-encompassing pankration in great depth, in addition to weapons competition (hoplomachia).

Topics include arms and armor, the phalanx formation, the pyrrich war dances, tournament rules, a functional analysis of techniques, and training methods along with a complete listing of all the Olympic combat sports champions from their inception in 708 B.C. until the last documented contest on record.

$24.95

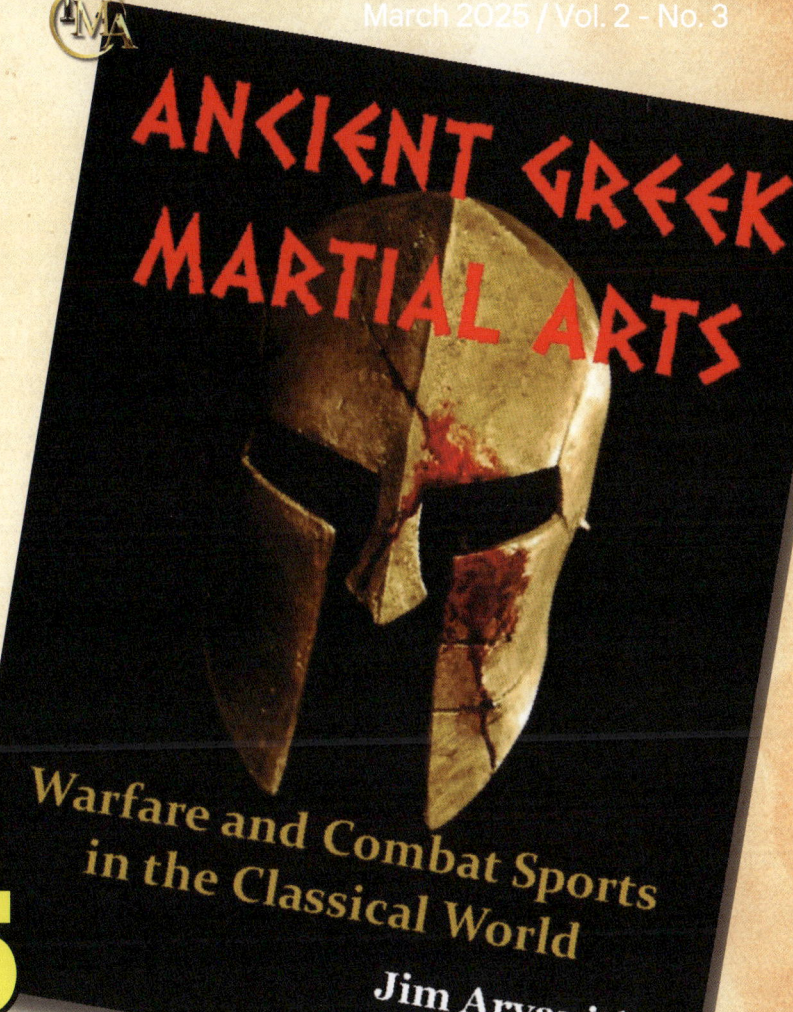

Emphasis is given to the role that combat played in Hellenic culture and its spiritual connection to the gods themselves. The book features photos of modern-day reenactors demonstrating hoplite skills and numerous works of art depicted on vases, architectural friezes, frescoes, sculptures, and coins showing combat athletes in heated action. A comprehensive glossary of relevant military and sport terms is also included.

AVAILABLE ON AMAZON.COM

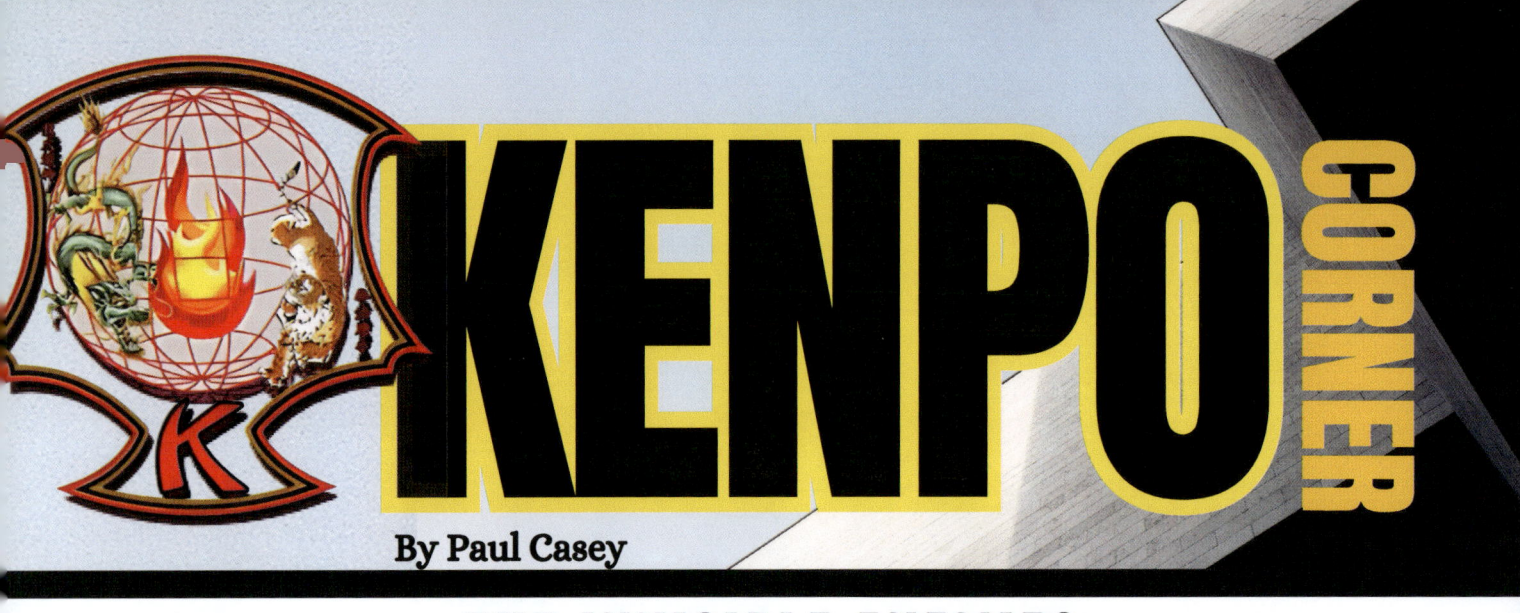

KENPO CORNER

By Paul Casey

THE INVISIBLE ENEMIES

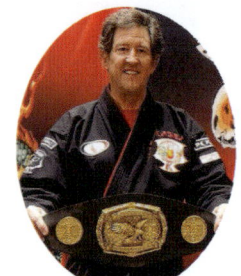

The key to one's martial arts journey is based on 'basics' or fundamentals.

There are three aspects. Mental, physical and spiritual,, which holds it all together. You must recognize them and seek training in them. The mind and body must work together. These principles apply in combat, and in life.

Balance is necessary.

Seek it.

Once you understand, you will strengthen your mind, body and spirit, and your journey will reveal itself.

Enemies will present themselves. Some are seen. And some are not.

Be wise.

There are eight considerations in Kenpo. Mental analysis will assist and prepare you, as time on the mat will develop physical skill.

Life's greatest battles are not fought with fists or weapons but within the mind.

True mastery of combat begins by defeating the enemies you cannot see.

Whether in the school, the ring, the streets, or the business environment, these unseen forces will either control you or be controlled by you. So, what are the mindset challenges?

Fear – Fear is the first opponent. It paralyzes action and makes you hesitate. In battle, hesitation is defeat.

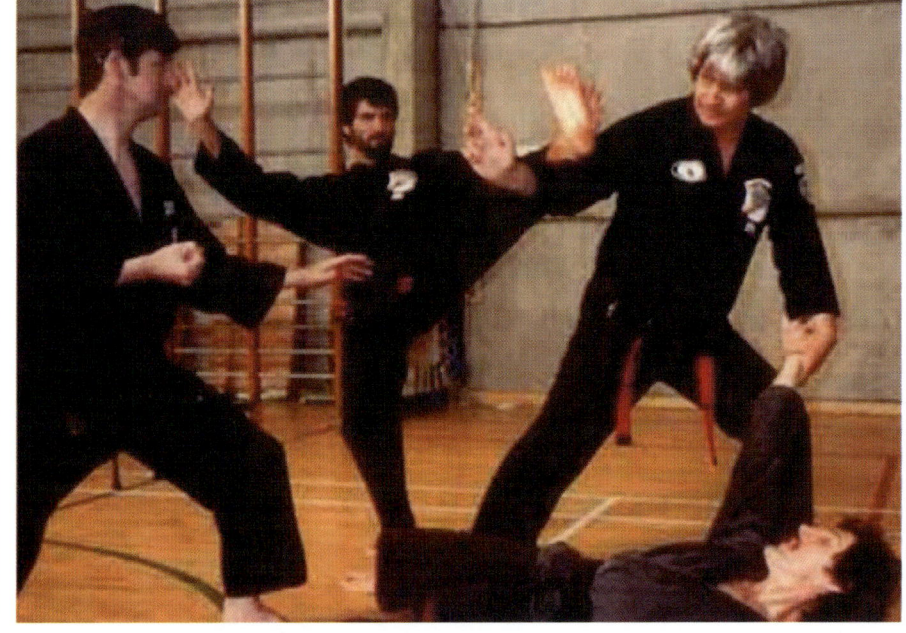

May 2025 / Vol. 2 - No. 5

Acknowledge it, then act despite it. Courage is not the absence of fear but the mastery of it.

Fear is a negative causing doubt. e.g. 'I cannot do this, or I will fail.'

Anger is a negative-positive. It heightens your senses but must be controlled with a calm mind. e.g., hot water in a pot.

Finally, Rage is a negative-negative which is uncontrolled. e.g. boiling water spilling out.

Turn 'fear' into controlled anger. e.g., an animal running away vs. a protective animal growling.

Not a rapid dog ready to be put down.

Doubt – Doubt is the crack in your armor.

If you question your own strengths, and abilities, your enemy will exploit it. Train hard so that your body and mind trust your technique execution without hesitation.

'He who hesitates, meditates in a horizontal position.' Ed Parker Sr.

Worry – Worry is wasted energy. In combat, the only thing that matters is the present moment. The past is gone, the future is unwritten. Therefore, focus on what is in front of you. i.e make it happen.

'Be in the moment.' Mike Stone

Be in the moment?

What you do with your time will determine who you are…do not waste time. Make time.

Control your destiny. Make your decisions. They are yours. You will be powerful.

Those that doubt, will criticize. Those that laugh, will laugh. But you will succeed because you, yes you control your moment, and it will reflect in your future.

Negativity – A negative mind weakens the body. If you believe you will lose, you already have.

Cultivate a warrior's spirit—one that sees every challenge as an opportunity to grow stronger.

There is no perfect techniques. Because there are no perfect attacks. Just perfect execution by you.

Procrastination – Delay in training leads to failure in combat.

Train every day as if your life depends on it— because one day, it might.

'He who fails to plan, plans to fail.' Benjamin Franklin

Ignorance – The unaware fighter is already defeated. Study, learn, and remain a student.

The moment you believe you know everything, you have stopped growing.

Pride (Ego) – Ego is your greatest weakness.

Overconfidence leads to mistakes. Stay humble, always learning, always improving. A true warrior is never above discipline. Proverbs 16:18

The difference between arrogance and confidence?

One thinks they can do it. The other KNOWS he can do it.

Envy – Envy poisons the mind and distracts from your own growth. Your only opponent is who you were yesterday.

Focus on surpassing yourself, not others. Use others' success as an example of the opportunity that is there for you, too.

Rage – Rage blinds you. A furious fighter makes reckless mistakes.

Control your emotions—fight with precision, not rage. The calm mind wins the war.

Laziness – Comfort breeds weakness. Train when you are tired, when you don't feel like it, when no one is watching.

Discipline is the foundation of victory.

The most Destructive enemies are self-inflicted. Avoiding them is paramount.

Guilt – The past is a weight that slows you down. Learn from your mistakes, then let them go.

Remember, a warrior moves forward, never backward.

Hatred – Hatred is a poison that burns the vessel it is held in.

A warrior does not fight out of hate but out of duty, principle, or protection. Keep your mind clear. Thus, results sill be based on sound decisions.

Stress – Tension slows reaction time and clouds judgment. Breathe, relax, and trust your training. The mind must be like water—adaptable, fluid, and calm in the face of any storm.

There are always more enemies that you may confront. But fortify your mind first. Control that you can control. Then, carry out your action.

Be not afraid of failing, but rather embrace the challenge of overcoming it.

Victory awaits. Celebration of Greatness is certain. 'He who know himself and knows their opponent will succeed 100% of the time.' Sun Tzu

Final Thought:
The greatest battles are fought within. Conquer these unseen enemies, and no opponent in the physical world will ever break you.

Train your body, sharpen your mind, and forge your spirit into something unstoppable.

A true warrior Is not the one who never falls, but the one who rises stronger each time.

Time to train. Begin.

Paul Casey

ABOUT THE AUTHOR

Paul Casey is a 9th-degree Black Belt in American Kenpo and the founder of the Kenpo Karate Hall of Fame. He is also an Ed Parker Sr. black belt and represented over 200 of the greatest martial artists in the KKHOF. His lineage in American Kenpo is through SMA <u>Frank Trejo</u> and SMA <u>Dennis Conatser</u>.

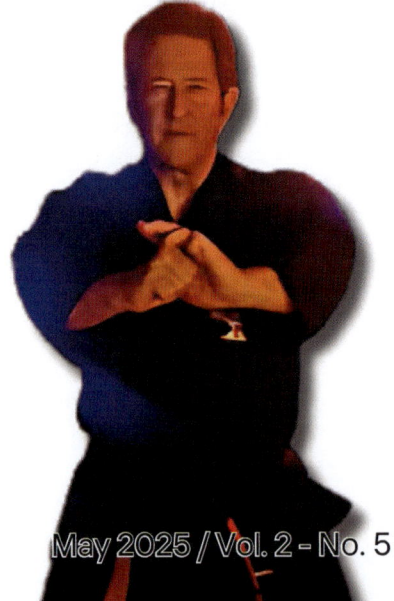

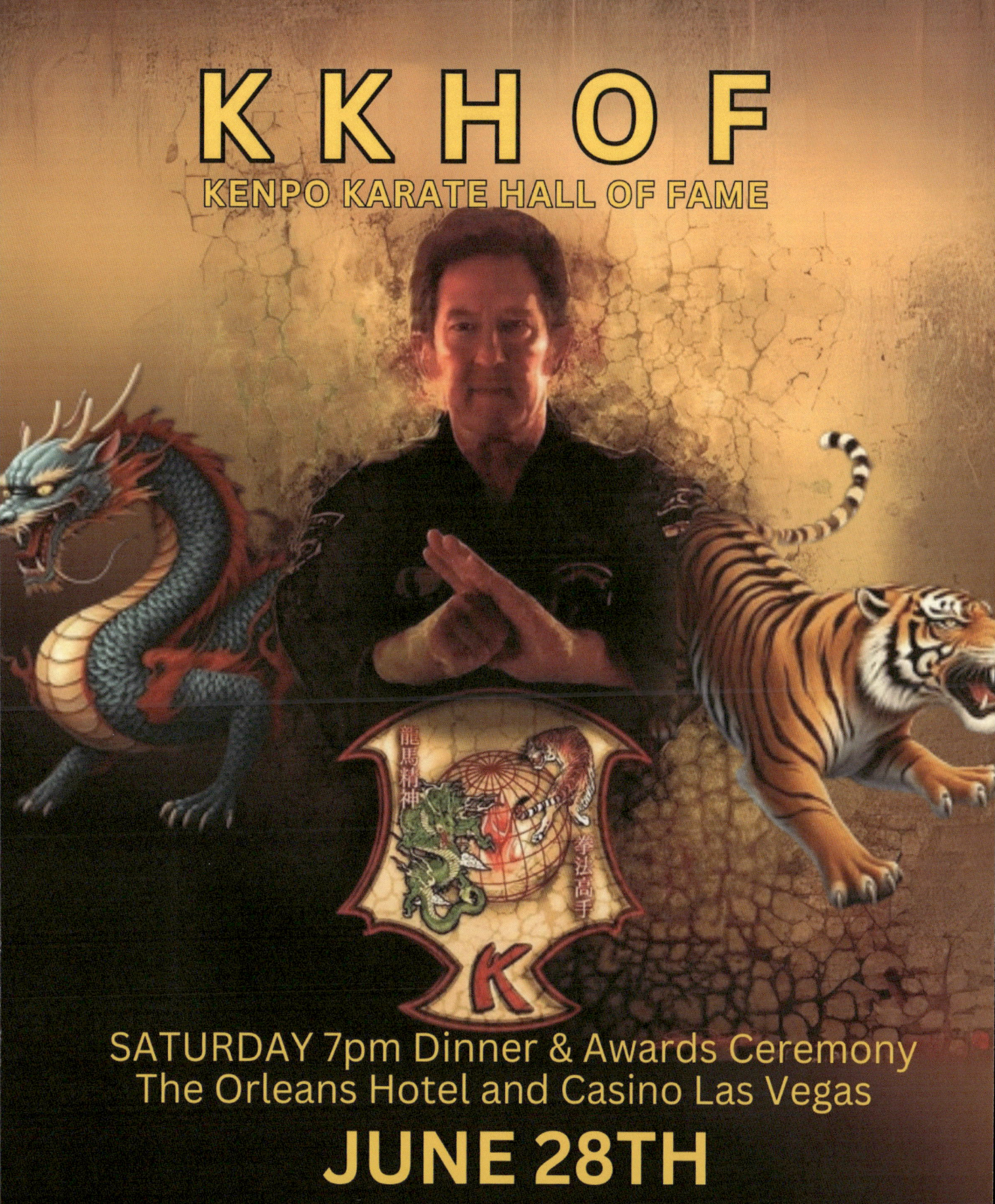

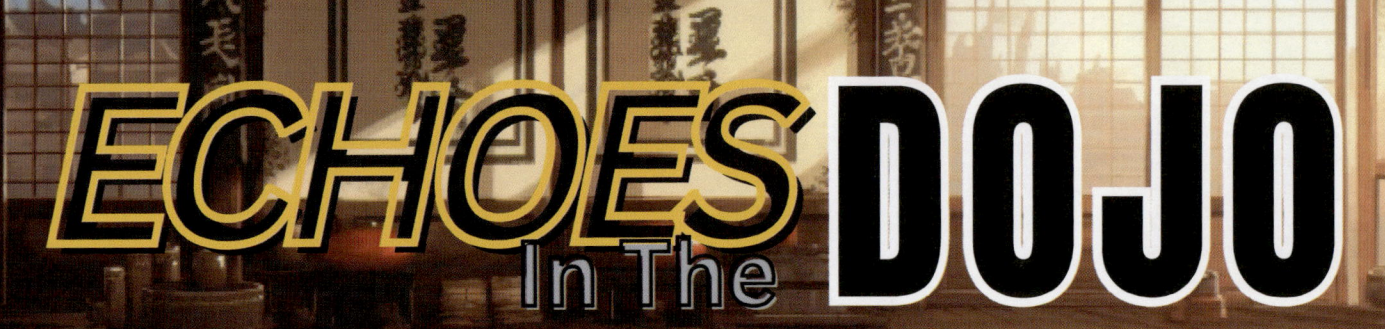

ECHOES In The DOJO
A MONTHLY MEMORIAL OF PIONEERS PAST
By Allen Woodman

RICHARD NORTON
A LIFE WELL LIVED

Richard Norton – A Legacy of Martial Arts and Cinematic Brilliance The martial arts community and the film industry are mourning the loss of Richard Norton, a remarkable figure whose life was dedicated to the pursuit of excellence in martial arts and cinematic artistry.

Born on February 6, 1955, in Sydney, Australia, Richard's journey began as a young boy, capturing the essence of martial arts and developing a passion that would lead him to become one of the most respected martial artists in the world.

Richard's martial arts journey was nothing short of extraordinary. He dedicated decades to mastering various disciplines, ultimately achieving black belts in multiple styles, including Karate, Taekwondo, and Brazilian Jiu-Jitsu.

His commitment to training and self-improvement exemplified the core values of martial arts: discipline, respect, and perseverance.

He was not just a practitioner; he was a student of the art and a teacher, inspiring countless students to follow their paths. Norton's impact extended beyond the dojo as he transitioned into the world of film. His career as a stuntman, fight choreographer, and actor began in the 1980s, where he made a name for himself in the action genre.

Richard's impressive filmography includes notable works such as "The Octagon," where he starred alongside Chuck Norris as a deadly assassin, showcasing his martial arts prowess and on-screen charisma.

His talents further shone through in major blockbuster films like "Fury Road," "Suicide Squad," and "Birds of Prey," and "Mr. Nice Guy" with Jackie Chan where he contributed his expertise as a fight trainer and choreographer, elevating the action sequences to new heights.

Beyond his on-screen contributions, Norton was a mentor to many rising stars in Hollywood.

His role as a personal trainer and instructor to actresses like Margot Robbie, Scarlett Johansson, and Charlize Theron highlighted his ability to adapt his teaching methods to meet the needs of each individual, ensuring they not only learned the mechanics of fighting but also embraced the spirit of martial arts.

His dedication to his students was palpable, as he instilled confidence and discipline in those who sought his guidance.

May 2025 / Vol. 2 - No. 5

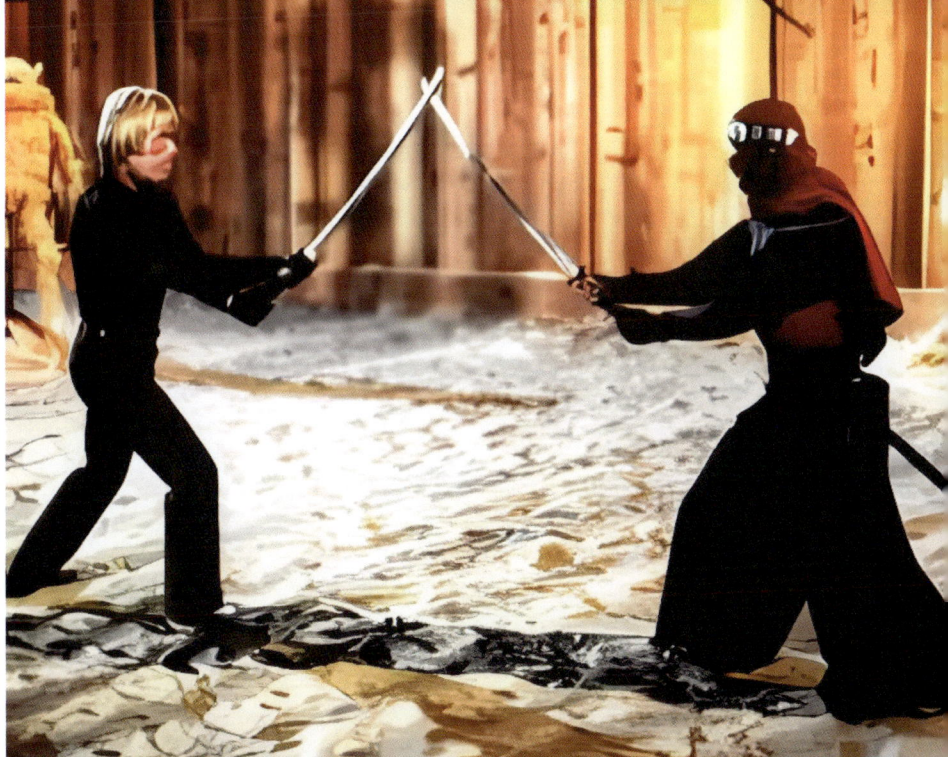
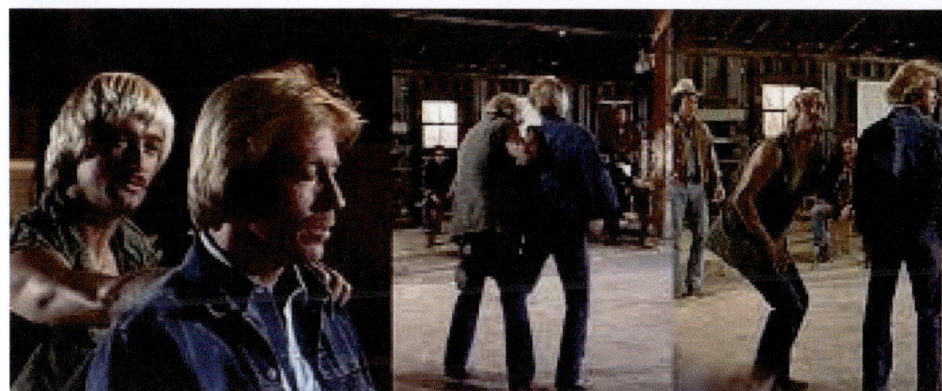
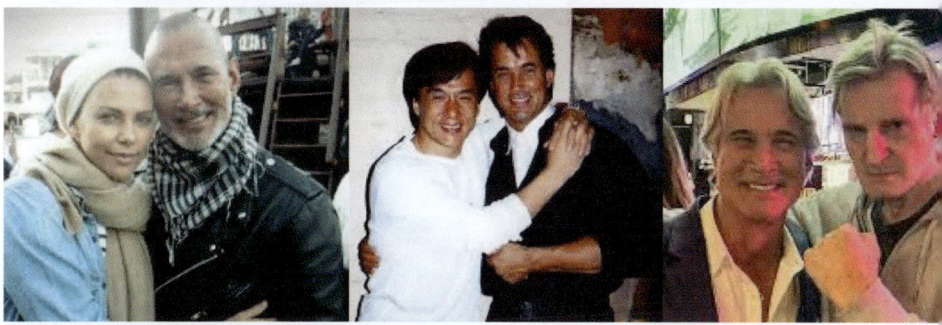
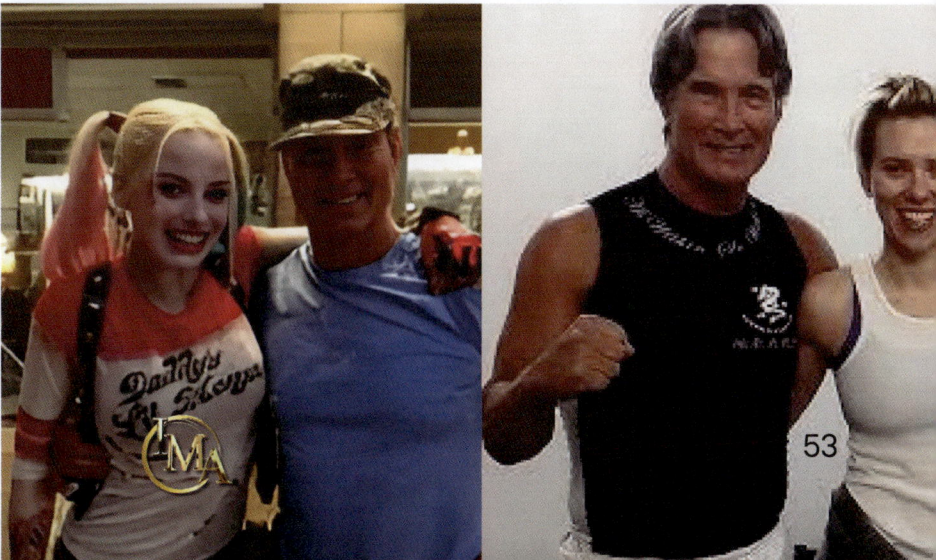

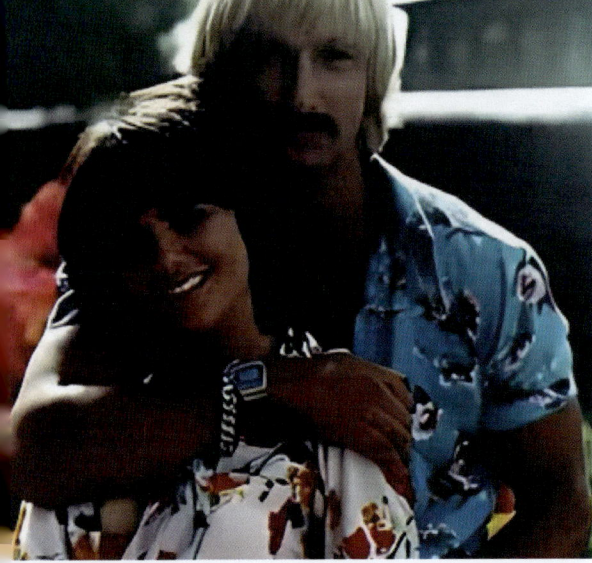

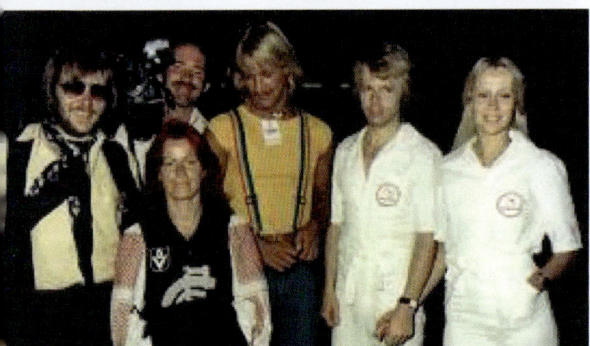

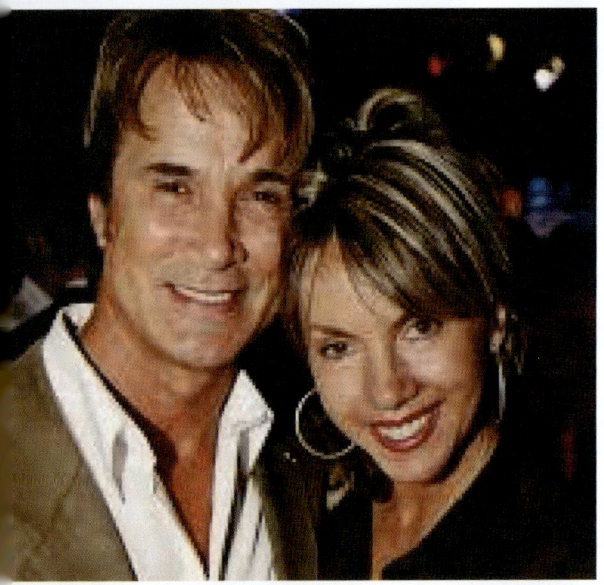

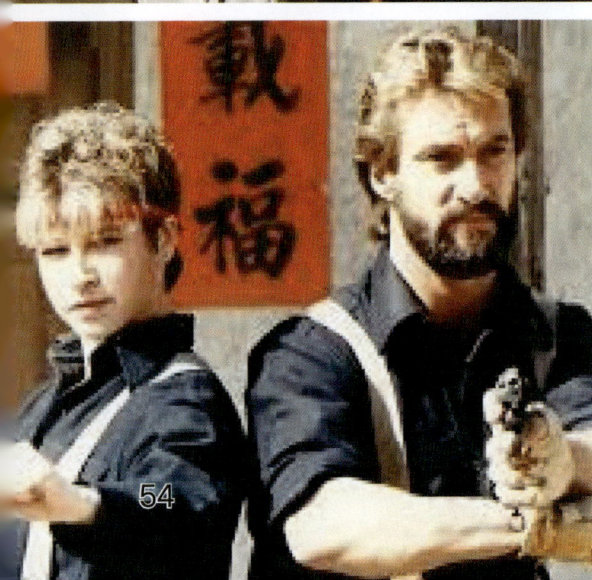

Richard's career earned him numerous accolades and recognition within both the martial arts and film communities.

He was more than just a martial artist; he was a bridge between the worlds of action and artistry, blending the technical aspects of martial arts with the creative demands of filmmaking.

Richard's contributions have left an indelible mark, inspiring future generations of martial artists and filmmakers alike.

As bodyguard for top Award-winning music artist and talent such as ABBA and Linda Ronstadt he always made personal relationships his priority and it was never just a job, it was a personal commitment to protect those close to him.

As we reflect on Richard Norton's life, we celebrate not only his accomplishments but also the spirit of mentorship and camaraderie he fostered in his community.

His legacy will continue to inspire those who walk the path of martial arts, reminding us that the journey is just as important as the destination.

Richard Norton's passion, talent, and dedication to martial arts and film will forever be remembered.

He leaves behind a legacy of inspiration, empowerment, and the reminder that with hard work and perseverance, greatness is achievable.

The martial arts world has lost a true warrior, and a personal friend for many years. His loss to those who knew him will leave an irreplicable void and his contributions will be cherished for years to come.

Rest in peace, Richard. Your legacy will continue to inspire and uplift those who follow in your footsteps.

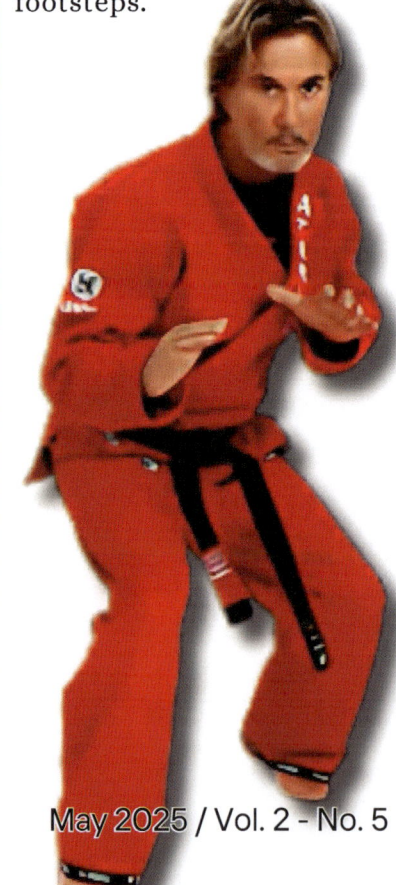

NEW LOCATION

KEEPING OUR HISTORY ALIVE

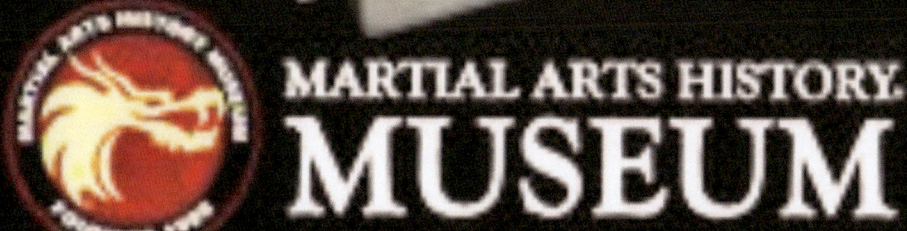

MARTIAL ARTS HISTORY MUSEUM

201 N. Brand Blvd., B100
Glendale, Ca 91203 (818) 478-1722
www.MAmuseum.com

HOJOJUTSU

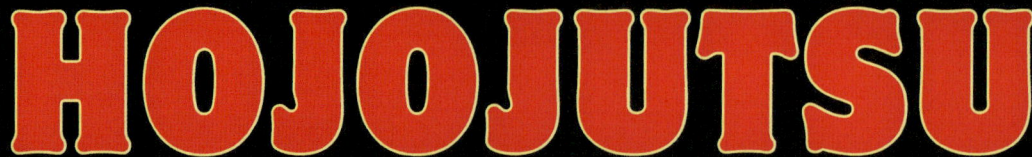

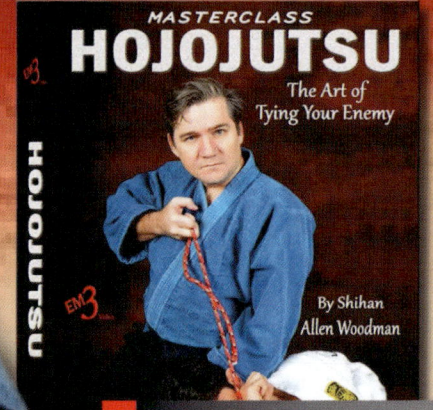

HOJOJUTSU
The Art of Tying Your Enemy
DVD 1
47 bmin.

$14.95
+ S & H

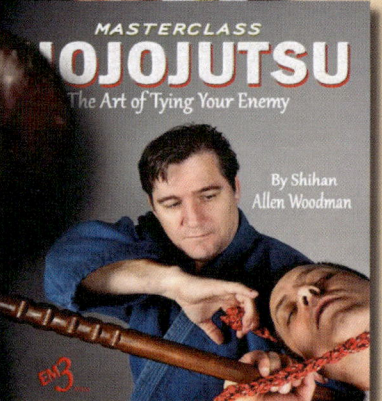

★★★★★

HOJOJUTSU
The Art of Tying Your Enemy
DVD 2
49 bmin.

$14.95
+ S & H

★★★★★

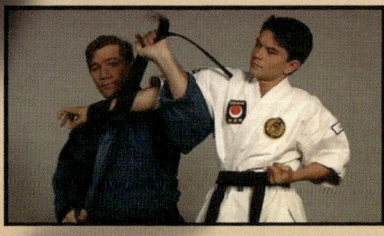 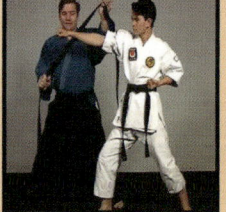

Step-By-Step Instruction throughout full color video

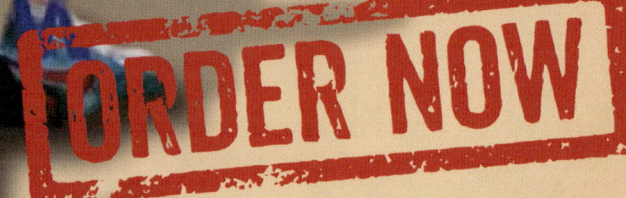

ORDER NOW

AVAILABLE ON AMAZON.COM
Available for workshops / Seminars / Events / Book Signings

BOOKS & DVD

Hojojutsu is a traditional Japanese martial art of restraining that encompasses different school techniques. It is a unique product of Japanese history and culture and is rarely practiced outside Japan. It is part of the curriculum under the aegis of bugei and in jujutsu. There are very few videos or books available on this art. Shihan Allen Woodman teaches you hands-on each technique in a step-by-step format.

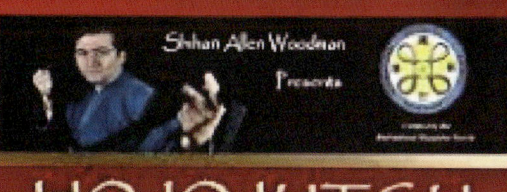

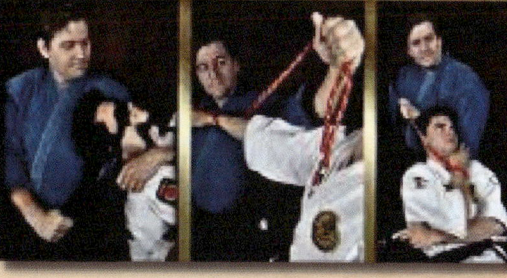

VOL 1 / VOL 2 $29.95 +S&H
FULL COLOR INTERIOR DIMENSIONS 8X8 132 Pages

★★★★★
Good information to add to what is presented in class.

★★★★★
New concept, for America, really effective

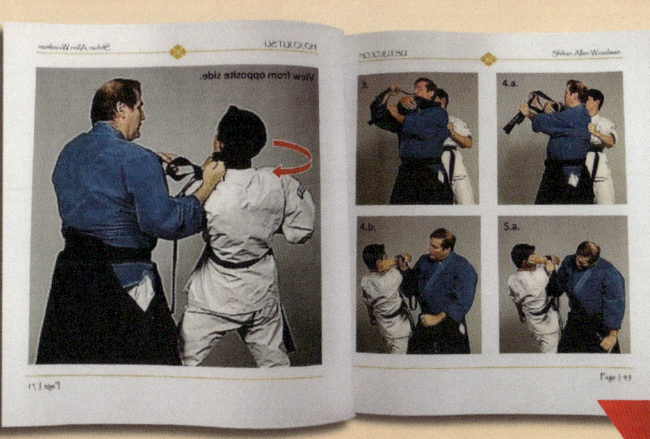

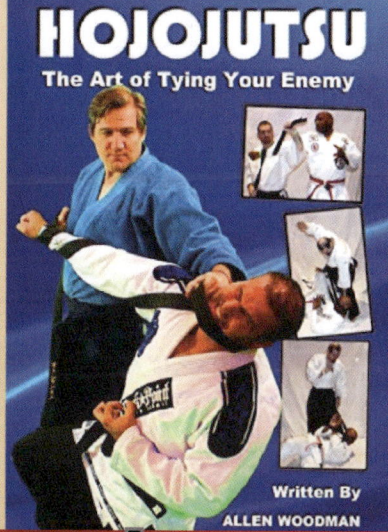

$9.95 +S&H

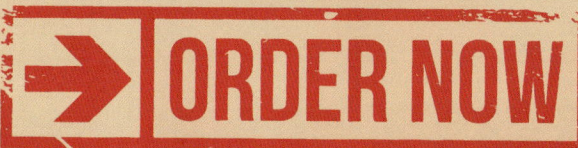
ORDER NOW

1 (725) 377-8092

allenwoodman1967@gmail.com

AVAILABLE ON AMAZON.COM
Available for workshops / Seminars / Events / Book Signings

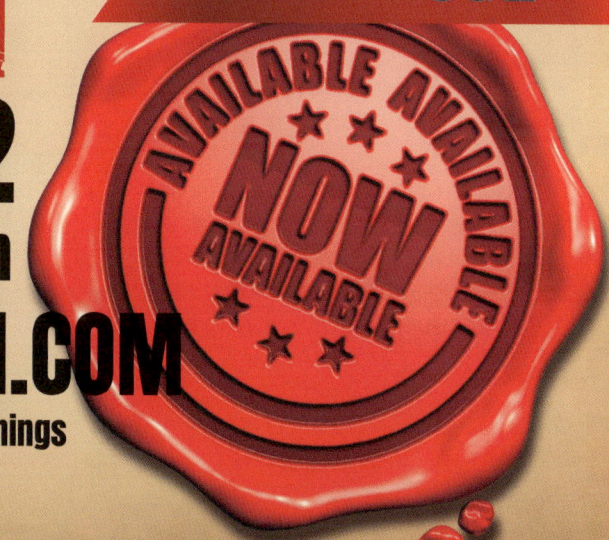

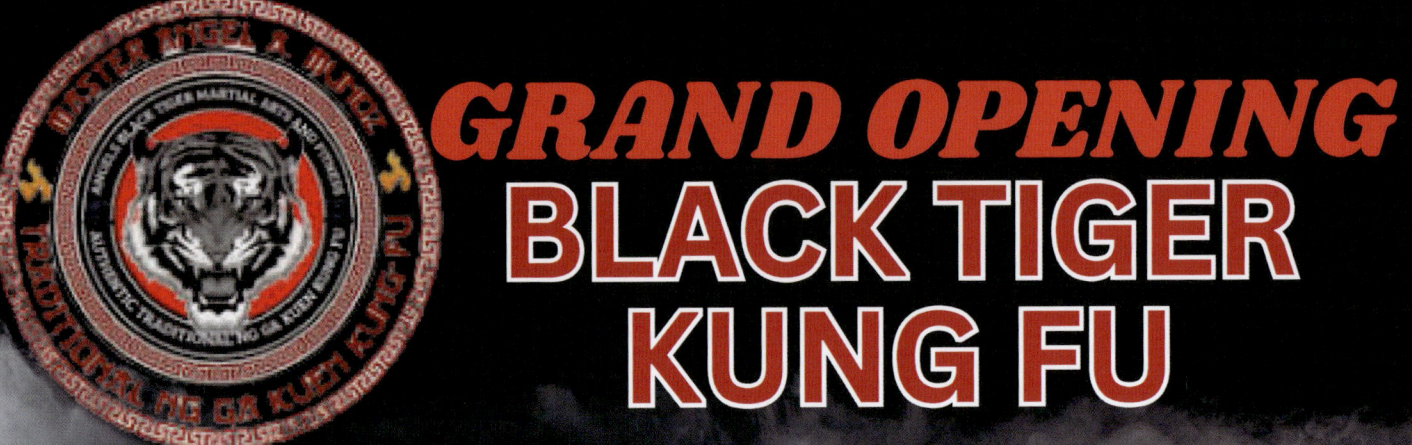

GRAND OPENING
BLACK TIGER KUNG FU

By Keith McCrary

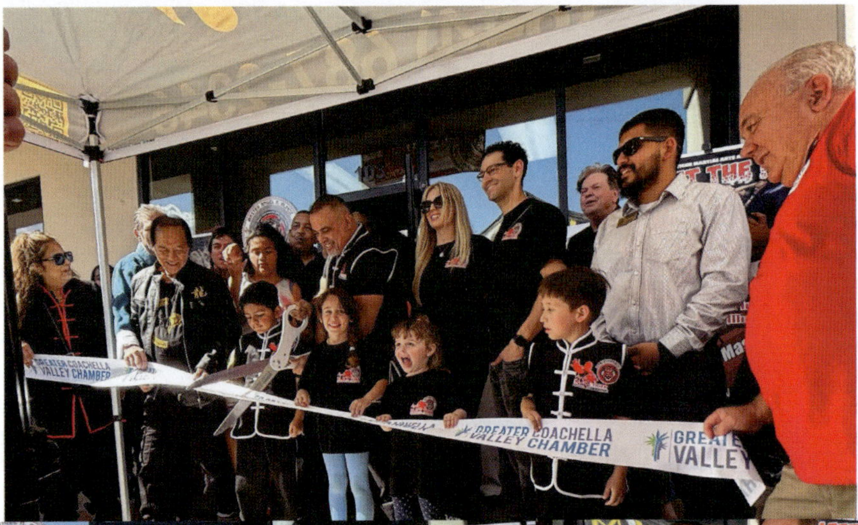

Palm Springs, California, recently buzzed with excitement as the grand opening of Sifu Angel Valazquez's Black Tiger Martial Arts school drew a crowd that spilled out onto the street.

The atmosphere was electric, filled with anticipation and enthusiasm for the new hub of martial arts training that promises to empower the next generation of students.

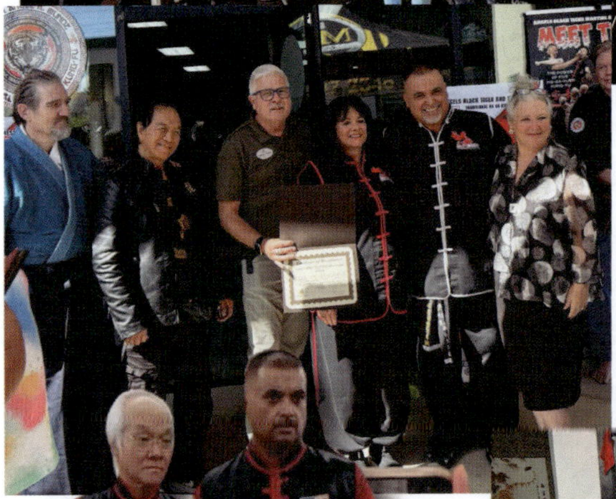

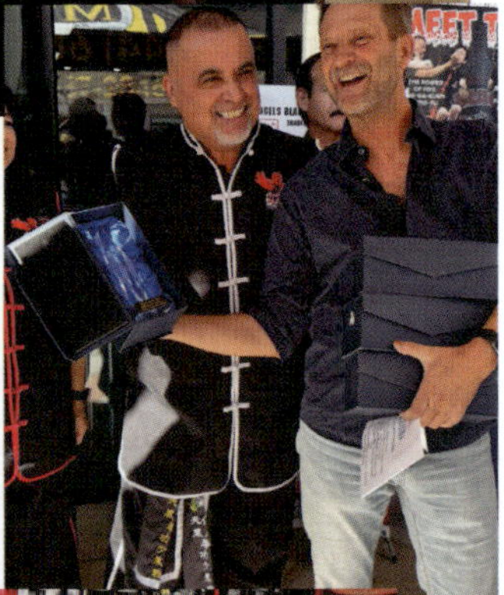

Sifu Angel Valazquez, who graced the cover of our one-year anniversary issue of International Martial Arts magazine, is known for his dedication to traditional kung fu and his passion for teaching. A direct student of the great Seming Ma.

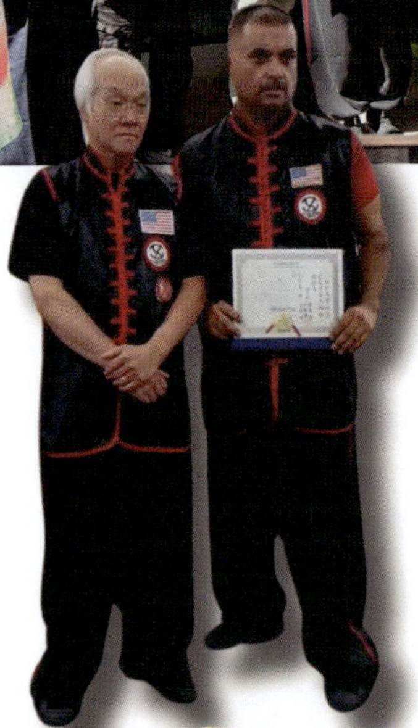

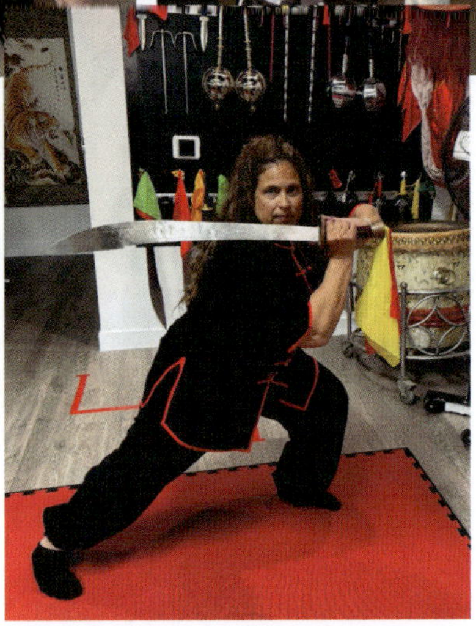

As the doors swung open, eager martial arts enthusiasts and curious onlookers filled the house, ready to witness the start of something special.

Among the notable attendees was our esteemed editor, Allen Woodman, who showcased his skills in a mesmerizing hojojutsu demonstration.

His performance captivated the audience, highlighting the depth and versatility of martial arts beyond the traditional kung fu forms.

Adding to the stellar lineup was Grandmaster Eric Lee, a five-time world champion whose youthful energy and skill were fully displayed. His kung fu form left the crowd in awe, reinforcing the importance of discipline and dedication in martial arts training.

Lee's presence was a testament to the strong sense of community within the martial arts world, as he joined other local martial artists in celebrating this new endeavor.

Other attendees included Sifu Nestor Moregon , Donald Hamby, Sifu Rosa Trenado, Vince Cicire, Jeff Powell, Mitch Shimer, Darryl Coneaux, Sensei Jimmy Willis, Elain Yamamto, Mike Zeggy, Jesse Dencil, Val Majailovic and Sensei Louie and Selina Palmer from Little Tigers in San Bernardiino.

The event was not just about demonstrations; it was a gathering of the community. Local radio personalities added to the festive atmosphere, while politicians and community leaders took the stage to honor Sifu Velazquez.

City Council members and the Mayor of Cathedral City presented letters of commendation and certificates of recognition, acknowledging his unwavering support for local businesses and outreach programs for children.

This recognition underscored the school's commitment to positively impacting the community.

Angel's Black Tiger Martial Arts is positioned as a vital addition to the Palm Springs neighborhood.

With Sifu Velazquez at the helm, the school aims to provide students with martial arts training and valuable life skills, fostering discipline, respect, and resilience.

As the opening day drew to a close, it was clear that this school is more than just a place to learn kung fu; it is a nurturing environment where future generations of martial artists can thrive.

The excitement in the air hinted at big things to come, and we eagerly anticipate the impact that Angel's Black Tigers Martial Art will have on the community for years to come.

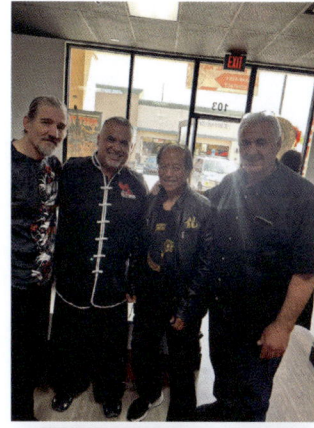
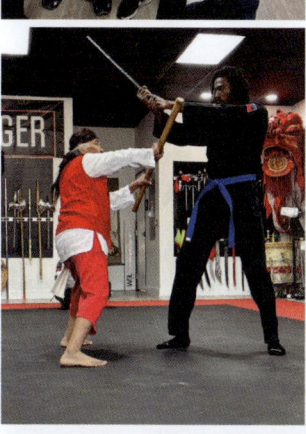
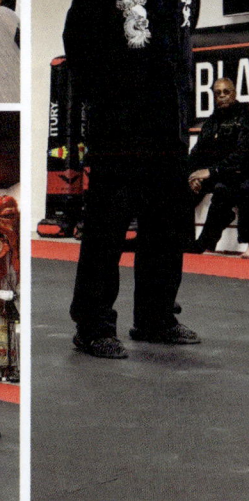
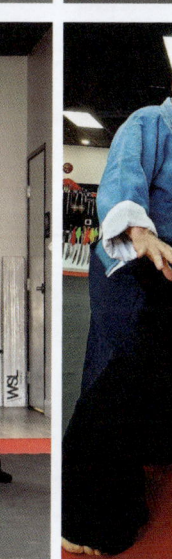
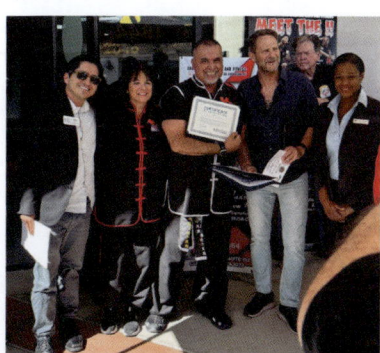
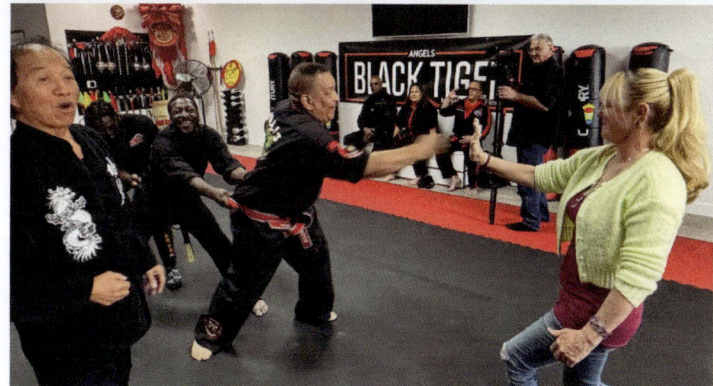
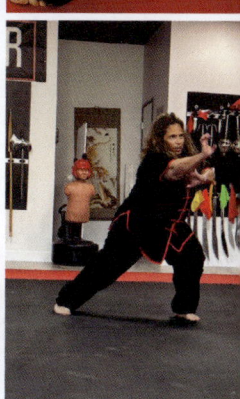

May 2025 / Vol. 2 - No. 5

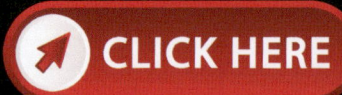

Printed in Dunstable, United Kingdom